QUIT SMOKING

Stop Smoking the Easy Way & Overcome Your Smoking Addiction for Life

(Guided Sleep Meditations to Beat Smoking Addiction)

Tyrone Stalcup

Published by Oliver Leish

Tyrone Stalcup

All Rights Reserved

Quit Smoking: Stop Smoking the Easy Way & Overcome Your Smoking Addiction for Life (Guided Sleep Meditations to Beat Smoking Addiction)

ISBN 978-1-77485-110-4

All rights reserved. No part of this guide may be reproduced in any form without permission in writing from the publisher except in the case of brief quotations embodied in critical articles or reviews.

Legal & Disclaimer

The information contained in this book is not designed to replace or take the place of any form of medicine or professional medical advice. The information in this book has been provided for educational and entertainment purposes only.

The information contained in this book has been compiled from sources deemed reliable, and it is accurate to the best of the Author's knowledge; however, the Author cannot guarantee its accuracy and validity and cannot be held liable for any errors or omissions. Changes are periodically made to this book. You must consult your doctor or get professional medical advice before using any of the suggested remedies, techniques, or information in this book.

Upon using the information contained in this book, you agree to hold harmless the Author from and against any damages, costs, and expenses, including any legal fees potentially resulting from the application of any of the information provided by this guide. This disclaimer applies to any damages or injury caused by the use and application, whether directly or indirectly, of any advice or information presented, whether for breach of contract, tort, negligence, personal injury, criminal intent, or under any other cause of action.

You agree to accept all risks of using the information presented inside this book. You need to consult a professional medical practitioner in order to ensure you are both able and healthy enough to participate in this program.

Table of Contents

INTRODUCTION 1

CHAPTER 1: SMOKING EFFECTS AND WHY YOU SHOULD STOP SMOKING 2

CHAPTER 2: THE SLAVE WHO CHOSE TO BE ONE 12

CHAPTER 3: INSTALLING EMPOWERING BELIEFS 15

CHAPTER 4: SMOKERS CRISIS 27

CHAPTER 5: DISTRACTIONS WORK (AVOID SMOKING TRIGGERS). 34

CHAPTER 6: TREATMENTS FOR NICOTINE ADDICTION 48

CHAPTER 7: GETTING SUPPORT FROM YOUR FRIENDS AND FAMILY IS ESSENTIAL 62

CHAPTER 8: SMOKING AND HEART DISEASE-THE CONNECTION 65

CHAPTER 9: MORE RECENTLY 75

CHAPTER 10: DIFFERENT WAYS TO QUIT 91

CHAPTER 11: BEST REASONS TO GIVE UP CIGARETTES/SMOKING 93

CHAPTER 12: RELAXATION TECHNIQUES 99

CHAPTER 13: MONEY 107

CHAPTER 14: HOW YOUR SMOKING AFFECTS OTHERS .. 134

CHAPTER 15: WHY PEOPLE CONTINUE TO SMOKE EVEN WHEN THERE ARE AWARE OF THE DANGERS ASSOCIATED WITH IT?.. 141

CHAPTER 16: BEATING ADDICTION................................ 144

CHAPTER 17: YOU'VE QUIT!... 149

CHAPTER 18: INSTRUCTIONS TO FOLLOW TO AVOID THOSE THING THAT MAKE YOU WANT TO SMOKE 158

CHAPTER 19: NUTRITION AND QUITTING SMOKING- MANAGING WEIGHT GAIN AFTER QUITTING AND THE ESSENTIAL QUITTERS DIET.. 163

CHAPTER 20: FOCUS ON THE BENEFITS OF SMOKING (HINT: THERE ARE NO BENEFITS)... 170

CHAPTER 21: A NEW KIND OF CLEANING 175

CHAPTER 22: HOW TO DEAL WITH WEIGHT GAIN AND OTHER SIDE 178

CHAPTER 23: CIGARETTE SMOKING CESSATION DRUG .. 183

CONCLUSION 193

Introduction

This book contains proven steps and strategies on how to finally quit that habit and have a better quality of life.

It's true what they say about smoking being a nasty habit that everyone should try to eradicate from their lives. There are so many ways and methods how to quit smoking but no one really takes that extra step to do it. This eBook will help you get your facts straight and hopefully you'll find it in your heart and cure yourself of that smoking addiction now!

Thanks again for downloading this book, I hope you enjoy it!

Chapter 1: Smoking Effects And Why You Should Stop Smoking

Effects of Smoking Cigarettes

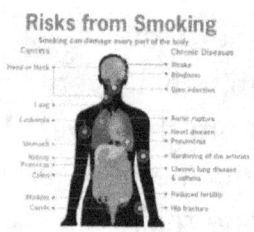

Numbing of taste and smell

Smoking cigarettes results in the smoker experiencing diminished sense of smell and taste. Doctors usually blame the numbing of the senses to smoking. This is actually proven when quitting cigarettes leads to the smoker experiencing better senses of smell and taste as well. A smoker will have problems experiencing the taste of food and other smells whether appealing or not. The diminished sense of smell is actually blamed for the accompanying diminished sense of taste. The fact that these senses diminish gradually means that cigarette smokers will not detect the same and will actually become acclimated to it.

Faster Ageing

Cigarette smoking is associated to premature ageing in smokers. Wrinkles, slim cheeks and stained hands and lips are just part of what to expect when it comes to cigarette smokers. Smoking cigarettes is attributed to constriction of blood vessels and the deprivation of blood to the skin. The skin ends up being deprived of the necessary nutrients and subsequently ageing faster. This ageing comes with the noticeable yellowing of the skin as well as wrinkling.

Impotence

Since cigarette smoking causes the constriction of blood vessels, erections are harder to attain and maintain. The blood vessels in the penis which are supposed to dilate for blood to flow and firm up the penis cannot flow therefore causing impotence. Young men who are smokers are affected by this problem. It is also true that cigarette smokers have a lower sperm count to pile onto the already alarming situation. For women, cigarette smoking causes serious fertility problems making it difficult for them to conceive. Women who smoke have to try longer to get a baby. When two smokers get together the chances of conception take a substantial dip.

The above are just some of the short term effects smoking cigarettes has on your body, it is however important to note that when you stop smoking, most of these effects including some long term effects as well reduce significantly and the body recovers with time.

When to stop smoking

With the above in mind it is possible that some smokers would want to stop smoking, however it is important to note that nicotine is a highly addictive substance which makes quitting very difficult. It is never possible to pin point when to stop smoking but it is important to stress that any time is the right time to stop smoking. The numerous health risks smokers usually expose themselves to mean that they can be reversed through quitting. This therefore means that whenever you decide to stop you will have made the right choice.

Most smokers have a problem quitting smoking due to the addictive hold that nicotine usually has on their body and brain. Their ability to function is limited when not smoking and constant compulsion and cravings make it even more difficult to stop. Cravings represent the constant bouts where the quitting smoker feels the urge to smoke after meals and/or during breaks. A compulsion on the other hand refers to the instances when the smoker is draw to smoking due to an unexplained feeling.

It is therefore recommended that smokers avoid quitting at a time when they are stressed as it is one of the main triggers of relapses. Stress causes cravings and compulsions to increase in intensity and hence increase the pressure that quitting smoker is under. When you decide to smoke it is best to have a support system made up f friends and family who can help you stay the course and cope with the pressure. However, note that relapses do not spell doom but rather offer useful learning opportunities. On average it takes a smoker up to 5 or even more tries to truly shake the habit and become cigarette independent.

A great way to help cigarette smokers muster the courage to quit the dangerous smoking habit is by educating them of the benefits of quitting smoking as a means of much needed motivation. Although some or most will ignore them, there will be some who will appreciate the benefits and use them as the necessary motivation to quit smoking.

Benefits of Quitting Cigarette Smoking

Apart from correcting the above stated cigarette smoking effects, when you quit smoking you also expose yourself to the following benefits.

Decreased Stress Levels

Research findings indicate that smokers suffer from numerous bouts of stress. Every time a smoker puffs on a cigarette after a few seconds they feel a sense of relief and their craving is satisfied. However this does not last for long and the nicotine in their system starts to drop and they suffer the effects of withdrawal although on a lower scale. This withdrawal is associated to stress, and until the smoker gets their fix they become stressed and irritated. By shaking the habit, smokers no longer have to deal with these episodes anymore and are happier.

Better Sex

When smokers quit smoking the effects of smoking including the constriction of blood vessels are negated. Increased blood flow improves the quitting smoker's sense of sensation and they get to enjoy sex more. This combined with attaining better erections means that smokers can enjoy sex even more.

Smooth breathing

Smokers usually suffer from regular coughs and labored breathing due to the effects of tar and toxic chemicals to the trachea and lungs. It is also known that lung capacity reduces in smokers by about ten percent. This may not be felt in youthful smokers who rarely engage in physically strenuous activities. However any time the smoker tries to run a distance they will feel the effects of this lower lung capacity. In old age, reduced lung capacity means that senior smokers find it hard to breathe smoothly even when conducting relatively easy tasks. Wheezing and coughing regularly can cause a lot of discomfort and lead to a lower quality of life in ageing smokers. This is easily eliminated once you quit smoking.

Higher Energy Levels

Once smokers quit smoking they feel more energetic and fresher on a regular basis. Increased energy levels in the blood do wonders for ex-smokers. The oxygen reaches all vital organs in higher concentrations leading to increased metabolism and higher energy production. Ex-smokers can enjoy engaging in physically demanding activities such as running as opposed to before. The increased oxygen levels in the blood with the reduction of carbon monoxide also help ex-smokers focus better and avoid regular headaches.

Smoke Free Home

There are many smokers who smoke in the presence of their children. Research findings indicate that exposing young children to cigarette smoke can kill them in infancy or lead to the development of various allergies and respiratory conditions such as asthma. This also leads them to think smoking is safe and can lead them to pick up the habit as well at an early age. Once a smoker quits smoking they no longer expose their families to the dangers of cigarette smoke. This is one of the most important benefits of quitting cigarettes. Ex-smokers save their children from the suffering the effects of smoking and hence give them a chance at longer healthier lives.

Chapter 2: The Slave Who Chose To Be One

Slavery has been abolished for a long time now, and yet, most of us are still a slave to something. I assume that the fact that you are reading this here right now, implies that you already tried quitting before but ended up going back to it. You probably even tried multiple times.

So when you smoke, who is really in control – you or the cigarette? Who is smoking who here? The cigarette is in control, you have made yourself a slave, you made yourself the puppet of a little stick of tobacco, the cigarette is your master, you are beating to its drum.

When you started, it was all good, you could have quit anytime. But you kept going. Before you knew it, you were smoking every day until the point where you didn't even have to think about it anymore. There was no real decision involved, it became automatic. It became a habit and now everything is on autopilot. There might be a cue, a trigger, an impulse and before you are even aware of it, there you are lighting up that cancer stick again.

I want you to realize and be fully aware of the situation that you are in. I want you to understand that you lost control, gave away your power, and that you have to reclaim it. Understand that you have been cultivating an unhealthy habit, by essentially investing in it, "practice makes permanent". The more often you smoked, the more embedded into your life it became, however, if you reclaim power, then reclaim your power again, and repeat to reclaim your again and again without backing down, you will return to that thrown of yours. You can become the master of yourself again.

As a matter of fact, when you quit smoking and become more powerful again, you will be more aware of other people that smoke and that pathetic habit. I know "pathetic" is a strong word, but in essence smoking is a reactive behavior that degrades us back to an animal level. Animals go by instinct, they feel impulses and act upon triggers that just make them do things. Humans, on the other hand, are able to understand their actions and the consequences involved, analyze their behavior, and then modify it. We don't have to act like victims. Nobody put us in our place and made us a slave but ourselves. If we made ourselves a slave, we can make ourselves kings again, it is that easy. "Life is 10% what happens to you and 90% how you react to it." – Charles R. Swindoll. Your time has come.

Chapter 3: Installing Empowering Beliefs

The starting point in the process is for you to believe that you can actually stop smoking. People using sheer willpower to control urges have success rates of around 5 percent, but the techniques described in the following chapters have success rates well over 50 percent. These techniques are far more effective in controlling the urges, but if you don't believe you can quit, they will be of little value.

Consider this analogy. Suppose two people need to climb a hill. One person believes they can reach the top. Even though they climb through the rocks and scrubs from the rough side of the hill, they will still be able to reach the top. Suppose the second person is shown an escalator that takes them to the top of the hill, but if they doubt they can reach the top, they will fail. Such thoughts as "What if the escalator breaks down," "I don't think I can stand for 5 minutes on the escalator," "When I step into the escalator, I will trip and fall," and similar negative thoughts will prevent success.

The techniques shown in the following chapters are like the escalator, but they will be of little use if you don't believe you can quit. What must be remembered is that even if you initially don't believe you can quit you can train your mind to install the empowering belief. If you are unsure whether or not you have the right empowering beliefs about your quitting program, just double-check your self-talk. If you think "I can't quit smoking because . . . I have failed a few times before" or "I can't quit because . . . I am not sure I can control my urges," these are the kinds of limiting beliefs that are natural for most people. It's because of past negative experiences or negative childhood conditioning, but these limiting beliefs can be changed through conscious effort on your part.

The two exercises described below can be used to install empowering beliefs. They work best if you use a journal. Writing your thoughts down on paper gives you a snapshot of your current beliefs. Going back a few days later and reading what you wrote allows you to see your thoughts from a different point of view. The gradual improvement in your belief system can also be easily verified by flipping through previous pages. You might need to spend a few minutes a day just going through the writing exercises before the beliefs are installed.

The following logical exercise uses past evidence to remove limiting beliefs.

1>Write down your self-limiting belief. "I can't quit smoking because I can't control my urges."

2>Then gather any evidence that suggests this belief is false. Can you think of other times that you have quit a habit? Can you think of other times that you ignored strong urges?

The second way to conquer your limiting beliefs is by using the "allowing statements":

1>Initial Statement: "I can't quit smoking, because I have already tried six times"

2>Follow-up Question: Has anyone else quit smoking after the sixth time

3>Answer: Yes

4>Allowing Statement: Thousands of people have quit smoking even though they failed at the sixth attempt.

While there are forty-five million smokers in the U.S., there are at least forty-eight million former smokers. When you use an allowing statement, you are basically asserting that since other ordinary people have gotten out of this predicament, so can you.

If you keep writing down your doubts in a journal and then keep following the logical procedures described above, your doubts will slowly fade away. You will get to a point when you will reach a sense of relief or a point where you will say, "I feel I can do this." This is the point where your negativity is being replaced by a sense of optimism and confidence.

These exercises are exercises of logic and don't rely on any visualization or metaphysical techniques. The most popular literature in the self-help movement concerns the Law of Attraction (LOA). The basic concept of LOA is "what you believe you can achieve." A great many classic self-help books have been written on the importance of empowering beliefs.

The following website has more than a hundred classic LOA books all for free.

http://www.law-of-attraction-haven.com/

If you are interested, I would suggest reading the following free books, all of which have sold millions of copies:

1>The Power of Positive Thinking by Vincent Peale

2>The Power of Your Subconscious Mind by Joseph Murphy

3>The Power of Awareness by Neville Goddard

If you think that it's just speculative metaphysics about beliefs affecting future achievement, please check out the work done by Carol Dweck. She is a Stanford professor who has done extensive studies on school children regarding the growth mind-set (her scientific terminology for empowering beliefs). Her studies show a remarkable improvement in children's scores when they have been trained to change their preexisting "fixed mind-set" to a growth mind-set. In the following TED-YouTube clip, she gives a great summary of her work:

https://www.youtube.com/watch?v=J-swZaKN2Ic

Once you are sure that the empowering beliefs are installed, the best way to quit is to pick a date when you are quitting. Have that last cigarette and announce to yourself that you are a nonsmoker on that date. You can write a small post-it note as a reminder and keep it in your purse or wallet: "On this date, I have decided to be a nonsmoker."

The six techniques to control urges described in the following chapters are NLP swish, NLP collapsing anchors, EFT tapping, Faster EFT tapping, mindfulness urge surfing, and hypnotherapy. Each one has been used by thousands of people to quit smoking. They are simple and easy to learn. Many people find a video demonstration easier to follow, so for each of these techniques, I have included a written description followed by YouTube links.

You just need to find one technique out of the six to help you control the urges. None clashes with another. If you find that more than one technique helps you, you can use the second technique as a backup if you become too bored using your primary technique.

All the urge control techniques discussed in the following chapters help you control your behavior after the urge has set in. They can also be used effectively to prevent an automatic trigger, which is something that induces an urge.

Types of triggers involve automatic triggers and emotional triggers—automatic triggers are environmental stimuli that induce the urge. When you see a cup of coffee in the morning, an automatic trigger induces an urge. Your surrounding environment will stimulate this urge, and your mind is conditioned to start smoking in that particular situation. Emotional triggers are usually related to stress. Sometimes, they could occur because of happy moments, such as social drinking. It's important to recognize and understand your triggers and how they set off your urges.

The automatic triggers can be effectively dealt with either preemptively or after the urge has set in. If you know, for example, that the sight of coffee early in the morning sets off an automatic trigger, as soon as you wake up, you can use one of the mind techniques to prevent it.

Even after installing empowering beliefs and finding a useful urge control technique, it's natural to be nervous about establishing a quit date. One great way to handle butterflies about your quit date is to set up "mini-quit" time blocks, which are just 2- or 3-hour time blocks when you try out being a nonsmoker. It's not meant as a challenge where you try to extend the time block. After the fixed time block, you are going to end up smoking. The purpose of having the mini-quit is twofold. First, you can test how your urge control technique does in "battle conditions." Second, your confidence increases that you can last a significant amount of time without smoking. If you succeed in not smoking during the time block, your confidence increases. If you succumb to the urge, you realize that your urge control technique needs to be tweaked. Either way it's going to be beneficial for you. Mini-quits are in effect rehearsal sessions where you work out the kinks in your technique and boost your confidence level. After several successful rehearsals at different times of the day, you will be ready to set up your quit date.

The amount of time you prepare before you set your quit date will directly influence how successful you might become. Scenario one occurs when a smoker just skims through this ebook, finds an urge control technique, and within a day goes about setting up a quit date. Scenario two is when a smoker goes about spending a couple of weeks installing empowering beliefs, learning stress-coping skills, and testing their urge control technique using mini-quits. The person in scenario two will enter the quit date with a higher chance of success. The more time you spend preparing before the quit date, the better chance of succeeding as a nonsmoker. The more effort and preparation, the better your chance of success is just common sense, but it needs to be emphasized that this principle also applies to breaking other habits.

Chapter 4: Smokers Crisis

For me, my smoker's crisis was borne out of desperation. I hated smoking, yet was a compulsive smoker. The more I tried to stop smoking, the more obsessive I became, the more I was convinced that my life would be lacking a vital ingredient for happiness: the ability to smoke whenever I wanted, especially at those special times: after a meal, after a cup of coffee, with a glass of wine. Those were the cigarettes I enjoyed. All of the others I hated, resented, and yet puffed away, even with a rasping, sore throat, just because I needed a nicotine fix.

When I gave up smoking, I was a single person with a high-earning job who did not have children, yet psychologically I suffered terribly because of my habit. Can you imagine the pressure felt by someone with a family on the lower end of the socio-economic scale, who knows that every packet of cigarettes they smoke are eating into their household budget, robbing their children of food, clothing, shoes, educational advantages and entertainment?

Smoking is a terribly inconvenient habit, especially now it is banned in so many places. Finding a place to smoke nowadays where you will not be a nuisance to anyone is not easy. Smokers congregate outside office buildings, and leave an appalling mess on the pavement; ash, butts, spent matches, not to mention the smell. They also gather outside bars and restaurants, constantly having to excuse themselves to feed their habit.

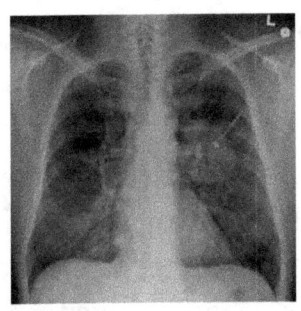

As a teenage smoker, I got into terrible trouble at school thanks to my habit. Smoking was strictly forbidden, and the penalties for getting caught were severe. It wasn't enough to stop me. I was willing to suffer dire punishments, especifically curbs on my freedom, in order to get a nicotine fix. The fact is, I began to associate cigarettes with sticking two fingers up to authority. This helped to deepen my psychological addiction in a very self-destructive way. Cigarettes have always been associated with counter-culture, rebellion and non-conformity, attributes that I wanted to associate with myself. I was very good at sports, especially at lacrosse and swimming, activities which are very strenuous and require high levels of aerobic fitness. This was not enough to persuade me to stop. In my twenties, I had an exciting career as a broker in New York and London. I used to deal with important institutional clients, and routinely made excuses during crucial negotiations in order to go and smoke a cigarette. This was fine when the clients smoked as well; in fact, more than once, being part of the "club" worked very well to my advantage. Smokers feel themselves to be a persecuted group who ought to stick together. This is a very powerful incentive to keep smoking, which we will explore in more detail a little further on.

My great-grandmother smoked until she was 89. She had a persistent cough and her doctor persuaded her that if she wanted to live "a long and healthy life" she should stop! She took his advice and quit immediately. Many people couldn't understand her decision, reasoning that she had lived so long, why make her remaining days miserable by quitting? Who wants to live until they're 90 anyway? Ask any 89 year-old, and you'll get your answer. She enjoyed her life and felt she had a lot more to do, and was persuaded that she would have much better chance of enjoying her remaining time without cigarettes.

Smoker's Crisis often involves fear. Fear is a powerful motivator. People who are diagnosed with cancer or emphysema are often so shocked that they immediately stop. The fear of developing these conditions is often as powerful as the actual diagnosis. How do you know that the next cigarette you smoke will not be the one that sparks off cancer in your body? My brother was the first one in our immediate family to give up the habit. He reached a point when all he could think about was how much he hated smoking and how much he wanted to stop. He caught a terrible cold, he felt lousy, yet he still continued to smoke. He was fully aware of how awful each cigarette was making him feel, but he "needed" the nicotine hit. When he smoked his last cigarette, he felt something tear in his lung. He was fearful, and immediately extinguished the cigarette, and has never touched another one. Shortly afterwards, he met his future wife, a nurse and a confirmed non-smoker. She sees only too often during the course of her work what smoking can do to people. She told me that she would never have gone out on a date with my brother if he had been a smoker. This story has a happy ending. He, like me, has no desire to smoke whatsoever, and they have two healthy boys. If he had persisted in the habit, his life would have turned out very differently. However, he has recurring sinus problems, which he is convinced is a remnant of his twenty year habit.

Chapter 5: Distractions Work (Avoid Smoking Triggers).

We are aware of the fact that smoking is an addicting habit and it isn't easy to quit this habit. When you are looking to stick to your resolution to quit smoking, you may have to fall back on distractions.

The urge to take one more puff can be phenomenally strong but the key thing to remember here is that it never stops with one more puff. You will find yourself taking one more drag and in the end, your resolution to quit smoking will go down the drain.

Triggers are the moods, feelings, places or the things that you do in your day to day life that turns on your urge for smoking.

Triggers might include any or all of these options listed below.

At the start of the day if you smoked starting your day.

Feeling stressed-while dealing with any problem or in stress, you feel like smoking

Being around smokers or smokes- when you are with your friends who smoke or with anybody who is smoking gets you into the urge to smoke.

While driving or in a car- while you are driving or in a car, you feel like relaxing or enjoying and feel like smoking.

After having a meal- when you feel without having a puff, you can't stay after the meals.

Drinking any alcoholic beverage- any alcoholic consumption is incomplete without having a puff to a cigarette, drinking coffee or tea when you feel like with these drinks a cigarette is so enjoyable.

While feeling bored-when you are doing nothing, you can be smoking. While you are over the phone, if you feel like smoking, then take a paper and pen and doodle to keep yourself engaged.

At the rest rooms or toilets- while you are at your waste disposal or in a bath tub, you feel like having a puff, without a puff, the bile's wont clear.

When a trigger hits, it's really tough for a smoker to resist the urge. Before you finally quit on the habit of smoking, you should make a point to learn your triggers and record them. Whenever you light up a cigarette, record the time, place, your mood, the company you are in, how intense your craving is at that time in a scale of 1 to 10 and what are you doing at that moment) when you have done your initial research, then have a plan ready to avoid those triggers as you don't want to get yourself into a smoking relapse once you have quitted.

This is why you need to take it slowly. Every time you itch to take a drag, you should try and look for some kind of distraction and leave your urge to smoke. Try and keep short time burst as you should delay the urge by say ten minutes. For the next ten minutes, try and immerse yourself in some kind of work. When you are busy and your mind is occupied, you are likely to forget the need to take a puff. Once you have managed to delay the desire to smoke, you should keep on postponing it until you cannot take it any longer. This is one of the best ways of curtailing the amount of cigarettes you smoke.

DELAY:

Delay the time of taking puff, when you can't stay on anymore with having a cigarette then tell yourself that you can wait for 5 more minutes before you finally light up, if at all you can't stop, at least doing this will at least reduce the number of fags you take per day at first. Repeat this process as often as you need it but don't stop doing it, result might be slow, but it will be there in the longer run.

Try and look for a type of distraction that can keep your mind busy and occupied. Distractions are the best way of taking cigarettes off your mind. The more immersed you are in your work; the less likely are you to remember taking a puff.

CHEW IT ON:

Have something while you are having an urge to smoke, just about anything healthy, any sugar free gum, or raw carrots, celery, sunflower seeds, something which is crunchy satisfying and non-addictive. You can also force your sub-conscious into false belief that you are actually having a drag. As you have something in your mouth, you will find that the craving for cigarette is likely to be less.

DONT HAVE JUST ONE MORE: when you have decided to leave the bad habit of smoking and have started the process of quitting then don't spoil your own efforts by having one more and then starting the process again, because it's only fooling your mind. It never stops with one more. And then may not ever get out of this fatal habit.

PHYSICAL ACTIVITY:

Physical activities can distract you from your cravings of having tobacco. Give yourself just half an hour daily when you can do moderate physical exercises or walking, jogging, if you are in the office stuck with work, you can take a break and can play your favourite physical games or whatever activity that interests you. If you are at home, do some cleaning stuffs, be with your kids, and play with them.

PRACTISE RELAXATION TECHNIQUES: when you feel like smoking, just that one more fag you feel like having. You can practise deep breathing or yoga or you can also try for some martial art. Relax yourself by getting a massage or going for safe hypnotic sessions. One can also try for some free hand exercises, or having deep breathing exercises.

GO FOR ONLINE SUPPORT: Join any online stop smoking community where you can discuss and share your feelings and problems with others. There you can see that you are not alone in your journey and that many more individuals are dealing with the same problems that you too face daily in quitting tobacco. There you can also share your success story when you have achieved some in your progress. You can also get important tips and helps there where others who are struggling or have left smoking share their experiences and success.

REMIND YOURSELF OF THE BENEFITS: Jot down all the benefits that you can think of in your writing pad and see them often to motivate yourself , or sometimes just say and rewind them aloud, amongst them one benefit is the monetary gain, if you spend say $2 per day on a cigarette packet then you are spending $60 per month and $720 per year and in 5 years you are spending $ 3600 and in 10 years you are spending $7200 on making yourself fatally ill and getting your medical cost more higher. So, all these add to woes and not to the benefits of smoking. So, point out all the possible reasons you can think of under the sun to quit smoking.

When you want to quit smoking, not only the methods but distractions also help you in your cause of quitting smoking. These are some of the distracting factors you may try while you are in your process to come out from this fatal addiction.

You can always listen to some soothing tunes or some upbeat tunes when you feel the urge to smoke, music can help you relax or turn divert your mind from the craving.

When you want to quit smoking, not only the methods but distractions also help you in your cause of quitting smoking. These are some of the distracting factors you may try while you are in your process to come out from this fatal addiction.

You can always listen to some soothing tunes or some upbeat tunes when you feel the urge to smoke, music can help you relax or turn divert your mind from the craving.

Play with your pet, when you are doing nothing and feeling like having a drag, then dog therapy or pet therapy as it is called may help to reduce the anxiety and the stress to have a puff or the pain that you are staying without a puff.

If you enjoy Sudoku or crossword puzzles then try engaging your mind into these games, or may be play chess.

You can also try surrounding yourself with people or in company of those whom you like or who encourage your cause or people who themselves are trying to get out of this habit, or you can call a good friend of yours and share a laugh may be.

You can also go to the gym and work out rigorously, you can also do some treadmills. Once in a while you can give yourself a treat, that you are trying to quit smoking and that's a commendable endeavour so if nobody does, give a pat on the back and enjoy a treat. That will boast your mind and confidence.

Surf the internet with your favourite sites on the list and see what's happening. Check on the latest gadgets and gizmos or may be gossip about your favourite star's life.

If you love your car, then wash them. Inside out, appreciate its beauty after cleaning, pat on your back on how well you have cleaned it that no other could have done.

Create a fund or an account and deposit the money you save daily from your smoking and reward yourself with that.

You can also indulge yourself into reading good books. you can go to the library to wind up some new thrillers or something that interests you. Library environment discourage smoking.

If you like bowling, then go for a bowling session, or may be a card game, or may be a game of squats. You can also go for swimming, or if you like photography then clean your camera and take photographs.

If you have a beach at your hand or even in a few hours' drive zone then go to a beach and enjoy the salty water with tender coconuts and beach volley, or you can also go to an amusement park and have fun.

There are many more alternatives and options on what you can do to avoid the instant surges or cravings of smoking. You just have to remind yourself that the urge or the craving will last for only a few minutes and you just have to win over that time. This is not going last forever either. If you can manage to quit smoking then you won't ever feel any urge or craving or pain like that anymore. You will be a free human being, Free to live a healthy and happy life, free from the fangs of this disastrous addiction.

These are all subjective methods and the results can vary from one person to another. Some people find it extremely helpful, while others may not be able to benefit from it. This is why you need to decide if it is working for you. Mostly, if you have an extremely intense craving and you want to have something because the lack of cigarette is driving you crazy, munching or chewing something can give you instant relief. Sometimes, it is not the tobacco that you truly crave for; rather it is the need to chew anything that drives you crazy.

These are all the common ways a lot of smokers have used for quitting their habit. Being distracted or occupied, both of them can help you out. Look for the kind of method that will help you out and then you can choose it to ensure that your resolution of quitting smoking ends up being successful.

Chapter 6: Treatments For Nicotine Addiction

There are many treatments available these days to help you break your nicotine addiction. They range from various medications to hypnotherapy. For a lot of these treatments, there is good evidence that they are more effective that quitting alone, or going cold turkey. The long term success rate for quitting cold turkey is approximately 5%. With the help of treatments for smoking cessation, the long term success rate for quitting can be as high as 30%.

Although a long term success rate of 30% may seem low, it is six-fold improvement on quitting without any treatments. In addition to this, it is important to realise that many people quitting on their first attempt are not successful, and these figures include these attempts. Treatments used for smoking cessation will be discussed in detail in this chapter.

Medications

There are several medications that can be used to help you quit smoking. Some of them are available over the counter and some not, and this will depend on what country you are in and local regulations.

Nicotine replacement therapy

Nicotine replacement therapy is perhaps the most common class of medications used for smoking cessation. These products essentially deliver nicotine to your system, without delivering all the other nasty chemicals that you would be exposed to through tobacco. The dose of nicotine can be slowly reduced until it is stopped. You may think that this sounds like a bad idea, as you are replacing one thing with another, and may become addicted to the nicotine replacement therapy. However the majority of harm from smoking is not from the nicotine, but all the other chemicals which you inhale. And although it is possible, addiction to nicotine replacement therapy is only rarely reported.

Nicotine replacement therapy comes in many forms; chewing gums, lozenges, patches, inhalers and e-cigarettes are just some examples. Each form of nicotine replacement therapy had its own advantages and you may find you have more success with one over another.

Chewing gums are ideal for people who feel they need to keep their mouth busy. Some people find the chewing motion takes their mind off any cravings they may be experiencing until the nicotine is absorbed. Chewing gum is also socially inconspicuous if you would prefer that people don't know you are quitting. Chewing gum with nicotine should not be chewed like normal chewing gum. It should be chewed only a small amount and then parked in between the gum and cheek. This is then repeated until the cravings disappear. The nicotine is absorbed through the buccal (cheek) and sublingual (under the tongue) route.

Patches also bring their own benefits to the table. They are applied to a non-hairy part of the body (ideally not directly over the heart) and can be forgotten for 12-24 hours. No-one would know you are wearing a patch as they can be covered by clothes. The site where you apply your patch should be regularly changed because if applied at the same site each day it is likely you will develop an allergy to the adhesive on them. When used patches are removed they should be stuck together (folded) and then placed in the garbage. This prevents the risk of a patch becoming inadvertently stuck to a child's skin. Patches come in 12 hour patches or 24 hours patches.

12 hour patches are applied in the morning on waking, and removed before bed. When they are applied to the skin in the morning, it takes an hour or more for the nicotine to absorb through your skin and into your bloodstream. They would therefore not be ideal for you if you wake in the morning with cravings or usually smoke within the first hour of the day.

24 hour patches avoid this problem. They are applied in the morning, and removed the following morning when you apply your next patch. These are good for people who have cravings in the morning soon after waking. The 24 hour patches however can, in some people, result in bizarre dreams and restlessness because

they are delivering nicotine to your brain when you are sleeping. This is a common side-effect and if concerning then they should be stopped.

You can even get pre-quit patches in certain countries, which deliver a lower dose of nicotine per hour and you can continue to smoke a lower amount of tobacco whilst they are being used. These may be usual during the time leading up to your quit date and some research has shown that they may boost the chances of quitting more so than if only using standard patches after the quit date.

Inhalers are great for people who feel they may be addicted to the process of smoking. By using an inhaler, you are satisfying the hand to mouth motion of smoking tobacco. You also obviously need to inhale from the inhaler, once again mimicking the natural process of smoking tobacco. Some people prefer not to use nicotine inhalers in public areas because of their look.

E-cigarettes are even more realistic, they look like cigarettes, come in similar packaging, the end may light up when you inhale as if it becomes hot and you will even find when you exhale that 'smoke' (a harmless vapour) will come out of your mouth. E-cigarettes are relatively new, however there is some recent research demonstrating they may be at least as effective as traditional nicotine replacement therapy. Until such products are approved by your country or states regulation agency I would advise against using these.

In some cases, it may be more effective to use multiple forms of nicotine replacement therapy at the same time. An example of this is where you can use a 24 hour patch, and then to use an inhaler for breakthrough cravings when required. If you think dual therapy may be suitable for you, you should speak to your healthcare professional who can advise you on safe options.

It is important to realise that all nicotine replacement therapies are medications and it is possible to develop nicotine toxicity by using too much. Using multiple nicotine replacement therapies together can increase the risk of nicotine toxicity. You should only do this when advised to by your healthcare professional. The risk of nicotine toxicity is also greatly increased if you continue to smoke tobacco whilst using nicotine replacement therapy. You should not do this except where strictly advised (for example, with pre-quit patches). Signs of nicotine toxicity include vomiting, sweating, tremor (shaking), palpitations (a sensation that your heart is beating fast or hard) and restlessness. You should seek medical attention immediately if you develop these symptoms.

Other medications for smoking cessation

There are other medications apart from nicotine replacement therapy available for smoking cessation. These medications work slightly different to nicotine replacement therapy and will be discussed individually. These medicines need to be prescribed from a doctor and cannot be purchased over the counter in a pharmacy.

Varenicline (Champix) is one example of other medication which can be used for smoking cessation. It is fairly commonly prescribed, particularly for people who have tried nicotine replacement therapy without any luck. Because the varenicline molecule looks like nicotine, it tricks the brains nicotinic receptors and is able to fit into them. This results in a similar dopamine surge as if someone was to inhale nicotine. One of the benefits of varenicline is that once it binds to the receptors, it binds so strongly that it stops nicotine binding to them. That is, if you are on varenicline and then smoke, it is likely that you will not receive any pleasurable effect.

The varenicline dose is usually started low, and then increased after a week or so to reduce potential side effects, particularly nausea and vomiting. Varenicline should also be taken with food to reduce any gastrointestinal upset. It is important to note, that because varenicline binds to nicotinic receptors in the brain, it is also possible to affect sleep in a similar fashion to nicotine replacement therapy. Varenicline seems to also increase the risk of depression or suicidal thoughts in certain individuals, if you feel this way then you should speak with your doctor immediately.

Bupropion (Zyban) is another medication used for smoking cessation. It was popular when first introduced but due to some significant side effects (such as suicidal thoughts and seizures), significant toxicity in overdose and other safer alternatives its popularity has declined in recent times.That being said, it is still used and may be effective for certain individuals. It is available as a tablet which is taken orally. The exact way that bupropion works is not well understood, there are theories that it may be related to its ability to reduce the brains uptake of dopamine.

Nortriptyline, traditionally used as an antidepressant, is another medication which has been used to help with smoking cessation. It is not commonly prescribed for smoking cessation. Nortriptyline should normally be taken at night time because it can cause drowsiness.

Other treatments available for smoking cessation

There are numerous other, non-pharmacological, treatments available for smoking cessation. These include counselling or phone counselling, support groups, acupuncture and hypnotherapy. Phone counselling services have been shown to be an effective way to increase the chances of quitting successfully. In addition to being evidence based, they are also very accessible for most people. Although some people may find acupuncture and hypnotherapy helpful in the quitting process, studies have shown that they are not effective.

Combining medications with other therapies discussed above is also more effective than either alone. For example, someone using nicotine replacement therapy who is receiving counselling is more likely to have success quitting that an individual using nicotine replacement therapy or counselling alone.

As you now know, there are many therapies which can be used for smoking cessation and it is important to tailor the treatment plan to your individual needs. The treatment(s) of choice will depend on many individual factors and previous successful or unsuccessful experiences with treatment. It is best to speak with your doctor or pharmacist to obtain individualised information and for guidance towards the most appropriate therapy.

Quit step by step

All the information provided in this guide may be rather overwhelming, and some people may struggle to know where to start. Below you will see a step by step quit process that is tried and tested, essentially summarising all the information in this guide.

Chapter 7: Getting Support From Your Friends And Family Is Essential

We all know how hard it is not to smoke when we're on a party, or just having a good time with our friends and family. It's very essential for your success to inform them about your decision and to get the proper care from them during the first couple of weeks.

During the years I've had a lot of friends struggling to quit the bad habit. They were doing fine until they had a couple of drinks, or we go to a club or something. I've found myself having the same conversation with every single one of them. It's important to have a trusted friend of family member to watch over you. Just like any addiction our mind is constantly trying to find a way around.

That's the time when we need someone to pull the cigar out of our hands, to turn the TV off when we see a character that's smoking or just to keep our mind busy so there's no time to think about it.

Speaking of someone watching over you...you should be aware and keep telling yourself that everything is for your own good and that you're better without them. I'm saying this because we all know how nervous we get after just couple of hours away from the bad habit. And nervousness can lead even to a fight with that dear friend who's trying to help us. This is why we need the constant reminder that we chose this, that we need this and we have to get through it.

For some people being alone during the first couple of days looks like a good choice but believe me, you'd want someone around you. Talking to a friend or family member can keep our mind calm, make us happy and believe it or not...happiness is a pretty good cure for everything. As long as we follow the decision we've made there's nothing that can push us out of the path. In my opinion every day during the first week is a struggle. I know what I want to accomplish and at the same time my mind and hands are searching for the one thing I want to get rid. But you have to know that you can do it, that you're strong enough to resist your own mind. After the second day you'll start feeling stronger, with more energy and a lot more.

Chapter 8: Smoking And Heart Disease-The Connection

Nicotine in tobacco expands pulse extraordinarily and pushes the heart as far as possible. Carbon monoxide enters the circulation system and replaces oxygen. Smoking likewise hinders the supply routes which may additionally prompt heart conditions and intricacies. Coronary heart illnesses are additionally predominant among smokers. The entirety of this ought to be reason enough for you to need to stop smoking.

Smoking cigarettes, as per clinical examinations, prompts a better capacity to burn calories rate and loss of craving. In any case, regardless of whether it is really loss of hunger or the taste buds losing their capacity of taste is vigorously discussed. The last might just be the explanation behind loss of craving. Directly after individuals quit smoking, they will in general put on weight. This could be on the grounds that their taste buds recapture their capacity to taste which makes suppers significantly more agreeable for the individual who doesn't smoke.

Smoking turns into a difficult one to figure out over some undefined time frame for an individual on account of the overwhelming fixation it causes. Nicotine enslavement is extremely difficult to beat; and one reason is that the synthetic compounds that arrive at the cerebrum from smoking actuates the joy spots in the mind. This influences the smoker's disposition and prompts momentary feel-great sensations.

Smoking Affects Sexual Life Too!

The vibe great sensation occupies the smoker from the way that smoking prompts lethal illnesses like malignant growth, emphysema and heart maladies. Indeed, even the sexual existence of guys and females, the same, are influenced from smoking. In men erections can be hard to accomplish and keep up. This occurs because of a few reasons, the essential being the job of carbon monoxide. At the point when Carbon monoxide enters the circulatory framework, it influences it by ruining blood stream to the penis. This is, as you probably are aware, required to get an erection. Smoking has been distinguished to be one of the essential purposes for erectile brokenness.

The Journal of Urology in 2000 discharged a report which expressed that around 68% of men with hypertension, around the age of 49-70 experienced erectile brokenness.

Among these, 45% included genuine sexual diseases connected to smoking. Hypertension is straightforwardly associated with low testosterone. Testosterone is a male hormone which has a tremendously significant influence in sexual excitement. It additionally prompts low sexual execution. Among other unsafe impacts, poisons in the cigarettes may prompt harming the testicles. Smoking may influence semen and sperm check. The portability and nature of sperm may fall apart. Sm

On account of ladies smokers, smoking may really hurt the ovaries. It is likewise hard for ladies to consider whenever they smoke and odds of imagining are decreased by practically 40%, during each menstrual cycle. So fundamentally, the more a lady smokes the less possibility she has of getting pregnant. Smoking along these lines unleashes devastation on sexual existences of ladies as well. It influences people groups' sexual experiences by lessening the nature of sex drastically in both genders who smoke. This is another purpose behind individuals to need to stop smoking.

There are numerous projects now accessible to the open which assist individuals with disposing of this propensity. One may likewise contact their own primary care physician to become familiar with the right drugs which can assist them with disposing of this horrible enslavement for the last time. These drugs normally wean the smoker off smoking gradually and dispose of the need to smoke through a timeframe in the end for good. It is an extreme procedure, however in case you're worried about your wellbeing, just as your stopping smoking is the best activity.

Stop Smoking Today!

Kicking the butt is viewed as one of the hardest mental tumbling one needs to do in the course of their life. Cigarettes are addictive due to the destructive nicotine regurgitating component it contains. Regardless of whether somebody figures out how to avoid the parcel of his most loved cigs every so often; nicotine withdrawal side effects begin to kick in. It is the withdrawal side effects that make it extremely hard for you to oppose the allurement of appreciating one more puff. All things considered, researchers have been diving further into the organic impacts of smoking and have separated a scope of mental just as physiological qualities which are liable for making us siphon on to this unsafe substance. Surprisingly, they have arrived at the resolution that by switching the elements concerned they may very well have the option to remove this propensity from a nicotine junkie.

Conceding your dependence on smoking

There is this regular propensity among most smokers to be trying to claim ignorance about their smoking connection. They reassure themselves by accepting they can without much of a stretch quit the propensity for smoking regardless of whether they know very well that in all actuality they can't. In the event that one at long last summons the mental fortitude to concede their dependence on smoking, the individual is one bit nearer to beating the smoking enslavement. When this acknowledgment sets, down the middle the fight is won.

Is it accurate to say that you are a smoker? It is safe to say that you are then embarrassed to be viewed as a type of feeble individual who can never get rid of his standard propensity for smoking? You have these senseless reasons like, "I need something to mitigate my nerves" or "It causes me think better". Reasons like "I have to loosen up" are likewise used to safeguard the propensity. Despite the fact that smoking is addictive, it's critical to not rationalize your propensity. Acknowledge that you have an issue, that is the first step in pushing ahead. Rationalizing strengthens that reality that you are unequipped for relinquishing your propensity in any case, and that you can't do any normal exercises without a cigarette. Concede that you are essentially dependent on smoking and attack the issue in earnest.

This acknowledgment isn't at all a shame, nor something to feel substandard about. Be intense and glad to stand apart from rest of the smoke-addicts. Tobacco is perilous to the point that it won't extra you until you capitulate terminally. Being up to speed in smoking makes no one can tell when you have at last let its savage grasp over you. It might be past the point of no return as it begins tainting every breath you take. You and no one but you can spare yourself.

The principal thing I recommend for you to do is to investigate yourself in the mirror. Take a gander at your picture in any event for a moment. Attempt to imagine the cigarette and its smoke as a lot of arms of a fatal octopus that has just grasped you from all around. It is maybe at this significant second that the acknowledgment would first light upon you that you are in reality dependent on smoking.

The idea may seem irritating at first; embarrassing on the main take. It might hurt your pride. Be that as it may, I disclose to you this isn't simply an opportunity to lose control. It takes a resilient individual to acknowledge their shortcomings. Try not to view it as something harming to your self image, rather marshal the fortitude to confront it. At exactly that point will you have the option to retaliate and recover your confidence.

You should notice this is no common fight that we are discussing. It's a hard fight that you need to battle until you win. Truth be told on the off chance that you adhere to the battle in the end you will win. Smoking will possibly beat you in the event that you let it beat you. You are the one that lights the cigarette; nobody is putting a firearm to your head. This manual will show you various techniques you can use to end your compulsion, in any case you need to adhere to the course of action to end to be successful. We can give you a guide to progress, however you are the one that needs to follow its headings.

Chapter 9: More Recently

More recently, I've tried to stop smoking, but the cure from Newtons Traditional Remedies is no longer available. More about that later, because about 12 years ago or more, I did find the solution to the very high cost of my smoking. And when I did, I wondered why it had never occurred to me before. At a stroke, I cut my expenditure on cigarettes to one tenth of what I was forking out, and yet I could still smoke as much as I wanted.

At the time I had resigned from the company I had worked for because new people came in and I didn't like the new set up. I resigned without finding a new job, which I figured would take me up to three months until a new salary started hitting my bank account. In the meantime,

I would exist on some money I had put aside. However, things would be tight and I needed to cut down and economise. The biggest proportion of my spending was on cigarettes, but at that time all thoughts of giving up smoking just didn't appeal. Yet, in the circumstances, I couldn't afford to.

I bought a pouch of rolling tobacco and some cigarette papers and tried to roll my own. It was a disaster at first because I simply couldn't get the hang of rolling a decent cigarette. As I tried to roll it, tobacco went everywhere. I then invested in a simple rolling machine, and some filters. Success! And I learned, through trial and error, that it was best if I dried the tobacco from its fresh (i.e., slightly moist) condition in the sealed pouch it came in.

At first, I was very self-conscious about smoking my own rolled cigarettes. No one in my circle of friends rolled their own. So I started out that I would smoke my own cigarettes at home and, if I was meeting up with friends or business contacts, I would buy a couple of packets of cigarettes. That was fairly short lived. I was getting used to Golden Virginia tobacco, which does not have any additives. It's just pure tobacco leaf shredded up. Conventional cigarettes have chemicals in them – quite a lot I've read. One of the main ones is saltpetre (Potassium nitrate) to maintain an even burn of the tobacco.

What I found within a short time of smoking just pure Golden Virginia rolling tobacco was that on those occasions I switched back to conventional cigarettes, I could taste the chemicals and the smoke wasn't as satisfying. Also, because of my ham-fistedness, I couldn't be one of those remarkable people I've seen who can successfully roll a perfect cigarette with one hand. I couldn't do it with two. I got myself a case and so I would roll 30 at a time and fill the case. And shortly thereafter, I didn't care if people looked oddly at me when I pulled out my case and smoked one of my pre-roll ups.

From a financial point of view, rolling tobacco is very much cheaper than packets of cigarettes. But even better, a quick trip to Belgium, and stock up with a kilo or two of tobacco at one third of the price of the same tobacco in the UK.

I mentioned the saltpetre thing because, whereas I was smoking on average four packs of cigarettes a day, in honesty I wasn't smoking that much. Certainly I was lighting that many and more in a day. But frequently I would light a cigarette, take a couple of puffs and then put it in the ashtray while I typed something on the computer or was distracted in some other way. After a while I would remember the cigarette and reach for it, only to find it had burned away. So I would immediately light another one.

With roll-ups, if I put it in the ashtray to do something, it simply went out, and quite quickly because it doesn't have any saltpetre in it. And so, I light it again when I want another smoke. In that way, the actual number of cigarettes I smoke in a day came down to 50+ on average, at one tenth of the previous cost of feeding my nicotine habit.

So for me, I had the freedom to carry on smoking as much as I wanted to, at a fraction of the previous cost, and I did. However, it is exactly five years ago, July 2007, that England became the last part of the UK to introduce legislation banning smoking in workplaces and enclosed public spaces, including bars. The days of getting into the smoking carriage on a train had ended several years before, as indeed had the smoking section of an aircraft.

At that time, with me just a couple of years off 60 years of age, I must confess that my smoking was impacting my fitness, through not doing much exercise and carrying a bit too much middle-aged spread were other factors. I didn't have a smoker's cough, but I would certainly get out of breath if I exerted myself.

In response to the new restrictions on smoking, I got very excited when I first read of it and saw a promotional video about electronic cigarettes which have cartridges containing nicotine. What an invention! And what a much better way to deliver the nicotine hit. No carcinogenic smoke and ash – an electronic mist of neat nicotine. A healthy way of 'smoking'.

I sent off for an electronic cigarette and a load of cartridges. According to the blurb, one cartridge provided about the same amount of smoking as just under a pack of 20 cigarettes. I was keen for this to work because it would solve so many problems. I figured I wouldn't be out of breath so much after a while on these things. They were perfectly legal to use in places where smoking was now banned because they contained neither tobacco nor a flame, and so were exempt from the legal restrictions.

My high expectations of this new way of smoking ended in disappointment. Great in theory but, again, the nicotine hit just didn't come up to scratch for a chain-smoker like me. And the claim of a cartridge being equivalent to about 16 normal cigarettes – well, if that was true, I was smoking the equivalent of 200 a day, because I found that after what, for me and the way I pull on a cigarette, would have been six cigarettes, the cartridge was wasted and I was sucking for all I was worth and getting hardly anything by way of nicotine.

Having said that, the electronic cigarette idea worked well in long meetings. As I said, legally, it is not smoking so I could happily do it, albeit to some disapproving looks, in a company meeting and elsewhere. But even then, it was a poor substitute for a proper cigarette, but at least I could last a meeting without being driven to distraction with my nicotine cravings.

I should mention that our office became a no smoking environment a few years before the legal ban and I approved of that. What I didn't approve of was how smoking disrupted my working day. I would arrive for work in the morning and stand outside for 10 minutes or so, topping up on my nicotine levels before entering the building and getting the lift up to the 7th floor where my office was. Within an hour, I would need to go back down and out of the building to have a smoke. And while I was there, I would smoke a second in succession, to try to make the gap to when I next needed a nicotine shot a bit longer. So, a ciggie break was about 20 minutes. In each hour or so!!

That problem has been solved because, for the last eight years, I work from home and only rarely go to the office for specific meetings, usually less than once a month. At home, in my home office and my own environment, I can puff away to my heart's content as I work. So, as a smoker, I have been incredibly lucky.

My smoking has affected other aspects of my working life. I used to travel abroad for the company on business assignments, but for the last eight years I have packed that up. I do other work instead. I remember flying to Chicago for a conference some years ago. I bought some of that nicotine chewing gum to last me the seven hour flight, figuring it would provide nicotine and keep me sane until I could get off the plane and have a proper cigarette. It didn't. I was chewing away like mad, and ended up practically eating the seat in front of me. I was like a junkie on cold turkey within four hours, with another four or five to go and it took a supreme act of self-control to contain myself.

So, Nicorette didn't work, for me at least. On my next flight, to Boston, I had another plan. I bought three bottles of coke and a bottle of vodka. I emptied most of the coke out and replaced it with vodka in each of those three bottles. When I got aboard the plane, I drank all three and passed out and slept until two hours before touchdown. But those two hours were total hell. Of course, that bomb plot to blow up planes with liquids taken aboard ruined that scheme when liquids were banned from being taken aboard.

So I stopped flying, pretty much altogether. Four years ago, my brother died suddenly. It was only an hour's flight to his funeral but with the stupid security arrangements, and messing about getting your baggage at the other side, there is no flight that is less than three hours from the time you smoke your last ciggie outside the airport terminal when you arrive to when you get outside the airport at the other end.

Two years ago, I flew to an event in Amsterdam, one of my favourite cities. The flight was only an hour, and I had a new way of doing it. I took along my electronic cigarette. As I was walking to the boarding gate, an air steward saw me smoke it (this jet black device) and said, I've seen you smoking and it's not allowed. I said you haven't seen me "smoking". You have seen me suck on an electronic device that does not contain tobacco, nor is there flame involved, and so it does not come under the legal definition of smoking. The flight, short though it was from London to Amsterdam, was still a pain and the electronic cigarette didn't help much. I was absolutely gasping for a ciggie when I got to the other end and smoked about four in succession.

In other ways, life has been ruined for a smoker like me. Standing outside a bar in the rain catching pneumonia to have a cigarette is not my idea of fun. I remember an occasion when I was standing on the pavement outside a restaurant in the West End of London where we were having lunch. I couldn't help notice stinking black clouds of diesel being belched out of taxis and buses crawling past me. And yet, two passers-by quite pointedly sneered at me for standing on the pavement smoking. Clearly they felt I was destroying London's crystal-clear air with my fumes.

I love the hypocrisy! Smokers are an easy target to demonise and restrict. Put it this way: If you had your young child in a buggy and I came and blew cigarette smoke directly in its face, I don't think you would be wrong to hit me. Hard! Yet people push children in their buggies down the streets of any town or city and ignore the exhaust fumes belched continuously in their face by buses, trucks and cars just a few feet away. Or, you live in a town or city and it's a warm day, so you open the child's bedroom window a bit. All that carcinogenic crap is floating into the room.

Passive smoking? Standing outside that restaurant in a narrow street in central London having a quiet smoke between lunch courses, there was so much filth and pollution that it had to be the equivalent of actually smoking a full pack of cigarettes within about 10 minutes. Some years ago,

I remember approaching Tampa, Florida, in a car and from about 10 miles off, I was shocked to see a dirty brown haze of pollution enveloping the entire city.

And if you live in a European city, just look at this satellite image that I first saw a few years ago and which made a profound impression on me. You can pinpoint every major city in Europe by its filthy atmosphere. That's what everyone is breathing in, every minute, of every hour, of every day, whether they like it or not. They don't have a choice.

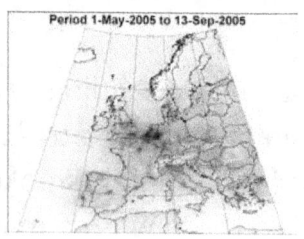

But I don't want to get on my high horse and go off on a tangent. Suffice to say I have honest, pragmatic, views.

Over a year ago I renewed my search for Newtons Traditional Remedies because I was ready again to stop smoking. It was because of the restrictions I've mentioned above and the fact that it was adversely impacting my levels of fitness. The catalyst though was because my second wife, after extensive nagging from her young granddaughters, promised them she would stop smoking. She's what I would call a mild smoker – about 15 a day. And, before Christmas 2010 she did take the plunge and give up smoking. The hard way. She was a tad irritable, shall we say, for a while, but she was determined to stick at it. She switched to the electronic cigarettes, but because they didn't satisfy properly, she had a hard time. But she stuck at it, even though the cravings for a cigarette were always with her, until she finally relented and eventually went back to smoking. Yes, she tried various techniques such as putting away each day the money she would have spent buying cigarettes and then, when she had accumulated enough, went and treated herself.

Before that, it seemed grossly unfair on her for me to continue puffing away while she was going cold turkey, but no way could I put myself through that. So, I just had to find Newtons Traditional Remedies and get my Lobelia cure. If I searched hard enough, I might find that although the company with that name had closed down, surely perhaps, someone from there had set up a new company. One way or another, I was going to track down a supply of those brilliant little white tablets that do the trick in just four days and don't involve any withdrawal symptoms or cravings. The easy, permanent way, or as permanent as I decide. My choice entirely.

Chapter 10: Different Ways To Quit

There are different ways to overcome your marijuana addiction. Three of the popular ones are:

Quitting Gradually:

When gradually quitting, the person reduces the amount of marijuana used, and continuously increases the intervals between each session. This is not a very effective method and has more chances of relapsing.

Quitting Cold Turkey:

Quitting cold turkey may be hard for some people but is one of the most effective ways to overcome the marijuana addiction. It takes a strong will and desire to quit that keeps the person from using again in the face of temptation.

Seeking Professional Help:

There aren't many facilities available for marijuana treatment, but there is professional help. The professionals help the person ease off and quit using the drug, and help alleviate the withdrawal symptoms with medications. Though, in turn, the person may end up becoming addicted to those medications.

In this guide, the method we choose as the most effective one is quitting cold turkey. Unlike other drugs, since the symptoms are mild and the addiction is more emotional than physical, there are no serious health risks when you stop using marijuana altogether.

Chapter 11: Best Reasons To Give Up Cigarettes/Smoking

The previous chapters of this book have been all about the horrors and bad things that smoking can give an individual. Fortunately, a beam of light now shines through this cloud of chaos. This is of course if an individual will choose to quit smoking. Smokers should never ignore the fact that these days, it is now possible to reverse many negative effects of smoking. In fact, good effects are felt almost immediately as an individual stops smoking.

Many websites and literature out there contain a wealth of information about reasons on why an individual should quit. Different versions of "quitting motivations" are accessible nowadays.

Actually, there is no need to be confused. One must just focus on the following:

Quitting for better looks

As stated in the previous chapter, smoking can make an individual look older, unappealing, and stressed. Yes, the body immediately goes on a "healing mode" when it stops receiving the poisons that are packed in cigarettes. Basically, the following benefits can be gained by an individual who stops smoking:

☐ The glow in the skin goes back to normal as circulation is improved.

☐ The teeth stop becoming yellow. Treatments to take off the stain on the teeth and gums become more effective.

☐ The breath improves in terms of smell. Even simple brushing and the use of mouthwash work in reducing or stopping tooth decay.

☐ The clothes worn by an individual will no longer have stains and will smell better.

☐ The hair and fingernails will show signs of improved health.

Quitting for Better Health

Health risks and diseases come with the use of cigarettes. These are decreased when one stops smoking. Below are some of the most significant health benefits that can be derived out of quitting or solving smoking addiction:

☐ Conditions of different body systems go back to being normal. Blood pressure and heart rates, as an example go to normal patterns.

☐ Taste and smell receptor cells grow back. This means that food will taste better and an individual can identify more scents. This makes life more enjoyable.

☐ Chances of developing different types of cancers go down. This also applies to other types of diseases linked to smoking.

☐ Medications and treatment procedures tend to work more effectively. This is the reason why even some forms of cancer are easily treated.

☐ The life span of an individual is generally lengthened. This is of course in comparison to the lifespan of a chain or addicted smoker. More years are added to the lifespan as an individual maintains a cigarette-free life.

Quitting for Loved Ones

Smoking is a deadly vice and addiction because it kills two groups of individuals at the same time. The user as well as those around him or her is affected. Others benefit from those who quit smoking as stated below:

☐ There will be no second-hand smoke that can affect other people. Inhaling this type of smoke is as deadly as smoking cigarettes. Those who choose to quit smoking give their loved ones a chance at a cancer-free life.

☐ Pregnant mothers will give their unborn babies a better chance of development without problems. Successful deliveries are linked to absence of cigarette smoke hazard.

☐ Those who quit smoking can be perfect role models for their kids and the people around them.

☐ Quitting and conquering smoking addiction with the help of loved ones builds relationships and solidifies personal bonds.

There are many other excellent reasons for a person to quit smoking. A long, healthy, and fun-filled life is not really that hard to achieve. Making the decision to quit smoking is just one of the steps towards this goal.

Chapter 12: Relaxation Techniques

Staying relaxed all the time is very important in battling the temptations of cigarette smoking. You will be able to think clearly with a relaxed mind, and your body will also become more resistant to the symptoms of nicotine withdrawal.

These techniques can help you achieve relaxation without having to spend a lot of money.

Breathing exercise

It was explained earlier on that the urge to smoke is actually a mere response to subdue the agitation caused by nicotine withdrawal. This agitation can be countered by increasing the oxygen supply in your brain, which is possible through deep breathing.

Controlled breathing helps in various ways.

First, filling your lungs with more oxygen ensures higher oxygen uptake of the blood and brain. The deeper you inhale, the more oxygen travels through your blood vessels into your brain. In effect, it also normalizes your constricted blood vessels due to cigarette smoking.

Second, higher oxygen in the bloodstream results to higher production of the feel-good hormones serotonin, dopamine, and oxytocin. These hormones do not only calm your senses and make you more optimistic; they also lessen the impact of withdrawal symptoms.

Third, a few minutes of breathing exercises has been discovered to stimulate higher production of endorphin, a feel-good hormone that also works as a natural pain reliever. This can help you manage and tolerate many symptoms of smoking cessation, such as headaches and muscle spasms.

Lastly, controlled breathing lowers blood pressure. This can help you calm down faster. Also, you should know that the strongest urge to smoke kicks in as your blood pressure shoots up.

So, are you already convinced about the benefits of controlled breathing when it comes to smoking cessation? But how do you do it exactly? You can do the following:

5-2-5 Rule — This is the simplest breathing exercise. The numbers mean slowly inhaling for five seconds, holding it for two seconds, and slowly exhaling for another five seconds. Repeat this over and over until your heartbeat normalizes and your senses calm down.

Equal Breathing (Sama Vritti) — This technique gives equal emphasis to the inhalation and exhalation. Inhale for four seconds and exhale immediately for four seconds. As your lung capacity improves, extend the length of breathing to five seconds, and then six seconds (the normal breathing count of yogis).

Abdominal Breathing Technique – This maintenance breathing technique aims to suppress or greatly reduce the urge to smoke. Done for at least 10 minutes a day, it starts your day by stabilizing your blood pressure and normalizing heart rate. Dr. Alison McConnell, a breathing expert, says that doing this for two months can make you feel the benefits longer.

Two-way/Progressive Breathing – In yoga, two-way breathing is said to be more effective in inducing relaxation. This is done by breathing in through the nose, holding it for two seconds, and then breathing out through the mouth. As you progress with this breathing exercise, extend the time that you hold your breath, ideally for five seconds.

Alternate Nostril Breathing (Nadi Shodhana) – This breathing yoga is said to balance both hemispheres of the brain by ensuring equal oxygen flow to both sides of the body. Yoga experts claim it to be an effective reducer of urge and withdrawal symptoms. It is done by inhaling through one nostril and exhaling through the other. Do it repeatedly and vice versa until you feel the urge disappear.

Progressive Muscle Relaxation

This relaxation technique is a combination of breathing exercise and muscle relaxation, which in effect calms the mind. This is the perfect relief for people who are feeling anxious because of nicotine withdrawal. It makes you more familiar with the sensations caused by relaxation by highlighting them against the feeling of tension.

It is also effective in releasing tension and relieving muscle discomfort. As the name implies, the technique involves different muscle groups, one by one, from head to toe or toe to head.

To start, lie down and relax your muscles as you apply the two-way breathing technique. Apply tension on each muscle group, and hold it for three seconds. Rest for another three to five seconds before proceeding to the next muscle group until you reach the last one.

Yoga

This Hindu system of exercises involves mental control and suppression of activity, done by maintaining different postures while incorporating meditation. This is a perfect way to induce relaxation while strengthening your discipline through mental control.

According to Mayo Clinic, people who practice yoga after quitting smoking have higher chance of quitting permanently. On the contrary, people who simply resume to their daily lives, without adopting any new habit after quitting smoking, have higher chance of experiencing relapse.

Habitually practicing yoga is one of the best things you can do to stay away from smoking for good because it trains your concentration and dedication. By controlling your thoughts and movements as you meditate while suppressing physical movements, you actually train your discipline, determination, and willpower. You become more in control of yourself every time the thought of smoking gets in your head.

Yoga is also an effective remedy for muscle spasm and headache—two pronounced symptoms of nicotine withdrawal.

Chapter 13: Money

Money should never be the primary reason to stop smoking. Health should be your number one priority. Nevertheless, smoking has become an expensive endeavor. Have you ever calculated how much smoking actually costs you? Most smokers focus on how much cigarettes cost them on a daily basis. A few dollars here, a few dollars there, who cares... Calculate it on a monthly basis! Check how much smoking costs you annually or how much you will spend on cigarettes in the next 40 years.

The average smoker smokes a pack of cigarettes a day. At the time of writing a pack of cigarettes costs from 7 $ in cheaper states and up to 14 $ in New York. Let's take an average of 10 $.

10 $ per day x 365 days = 3,650 $ per year = 146,000 $ in 40 years!

The number is very big, but that is not all. How about if instead of buying cigarettes you decide to invest all that money. You could deposit it in a bank account or even better in investment fund that invests in stocks. With stocks returning an average of 7% per year, let's calculate your opportunity costs of smoking.

Adding 3,650 $ each year in an stocks investment fund and letting it grow by 7% annually, how much money would you have in 40 years? Sit down. Are you ready?

A whopping 783,000 $

No, it is not a typo and I am not kidding.

How can it be? You will spend "only" 146,000 $ in 40 years, so where does additional 600,000 $ come from? That is compounding and yes, it works like magic. The longer your horizon, the longer your money earns interest for you. If you leave the money in the fund, interests you receive also earn interests. That is why in 40 years the money in the fund grows more than 500 %. Check the table below to see the calculation and to see how compounding is making you richer and richer each year. That is your smoking opportunity cost. If you choose to smoke, you give up all this money. 7 % annual return is totally achievable - that is how much stocks returned on average in the last 100 years.

Instead of smoking you, could retire to Florida, maybe buy a mansion in Thailand, beach house in Mexico, or a lovely cottage in the Swiss Alps. Heck, you could travel around the world for 20 years with all that cash. I mean, you can probably find a way to spend an almost 800,000 $, right? If you quit smoking you will also live and stay healthy longer, to be able to enjoy all this money.

If you check the table you will see that after 40 years, you get more than 50,000 $ of interest each year. Imagine what you could do with this money. Even if you smoke "only" half a pack a day, this still adds to almost 400.000 $ in 40 years. And if 40 years is too long horizon for you, investing 3,650 USD each year adds up to 160,000 $ in 20 years. No more excuses, smoking costs you a lot of money!

Time	Money added	7% return
Year 1	3.650	3.906
Year 2	3.650	8.084
Year 3	3.650	12.556

Year 4	3.650	17.340
Year 5	3.650	22.460
Year 6	3.650	27.937
Year 7	3.650	33.798
Year 8	3.650	40.070
Year 9	3.650	46.780
Year 10	3.650	53.960
Year 11	3.650	61.643
Year 12	3.650	69.863
Year 13	3.650	78.659
Year 14	3.650	88.071
Year 15	3.650	98.141

Year 16	3.650	108.917
Year 17	3.650	120.446
Year 18	3.650	132.783
Year 19	3.650	145.984
Year 20	3.650	160.108
Year 21	3.650	175.221
Year 22	3.650	191.392
Year 23	3.650	208.695
Year 24	3.650	227.209
Year 25	3.650	247.019
Year 26	3.650	268.216
Year 27	3.650	290.897

Year 28	3.650	315.165
Year 29	3.650	341.132
Year 30	3.650	368.917
Year 31	3.650	398.646
Year 32	3.650	430.457
Year 33	3.650	464.494
Year 34	3.650	500.915
Year 35	3.650	539.884
Year 36	3.650	581.582
Year 37	3.650	626.198
Year 38	3.650	673.937
Year 39	3.650	725.018

| Year 40 | 3.650 | 779.675 |

We are not done yet. How about if you add the money spent on buying "smoking equipment", lighters, matches and an occasional ashtray etc. The money spent on chewing gums and breath fresheners. Add the bills you pay at the dentist office to remove tartar from your teeth. Add other smoking related health costs. You could invest all that money too. Now we are talking what, a million dollars?

What would you do, if you were a healthy retiree with an additional one million dollars? It might sound like a fairy tale, but numbers don't lie. Most countries, including United States, are increasing taxes on cigarettes. That means smoking will become increasingly more expensive. Calculations above are for that reason on conservative side.

It is an illusion that smoking is not that expensive, because you buy cigarettes daily. Would you still smoke if you were to buy them only once a year? Would you go to the store with 3,650 $ in your pocket to buy cigarettes? I doubt it.

Ok, maybe you are not good at delaying gratification. Not all the people are prepared to invest money previously spent on cigarettes for 40 years. It does not matter. If you want to enjoy all this money now, why not fly to Hawaii at the end of the year. Imagine the sounds of the waves, the sun and cocktails on the beach. How about new bicycle you've always wanted? Or a beautiful dress.

There are countless healthier and more enjoyable ways to spend that money. Make a list of things you want to buy in the next few years. See how many things from the list you could buy with the cash you used to spend on cigarettes. If you enjoy inexpensive things like reading books, chances are that you will have trouble spending all that money. 3,650 $ is enough money to buy 20 $ book every other day.

Some ex-smokers like to put the money they spent on cigarettes in a special box. If you decide to do it also, you will be pleasantly surprised at how much money is in the box at the end of the year. Take out some money out of the box and treat yourself or your family with it. You have deserved it. It does not matter what you do with it, anything is better than to spend it on death sticks.

I suggest investing it and spending it later. Interests earned quadruples it in 40 years. Instead of 180,000 $ you end up with almost 800,000 $!

Step-by-step plan on how to quit smoking!

You should be ready to quit smoking and your motivation should be high! Motivation plays a critical role when you decide to quit smoking. It gives you energy and strength to endure.

Nicotine addiction is like any other addiction - hard to break at the beginning, then it gets easier with each passing day, until finally, you can't believe that you were once addicted.

Look, it will be hard at times. Anyone telling you stopping smoking is easy is lying. That reminds me of the famous saying by Mark Twain: "Quitting smoking is easy; I have done it hundred times already" That explains everything - staying non-smoker is the hard part, if you do it the wrong way!

In the next chapters, you will find a step-by-step plan to successfully stop smoking, for life!

No smoking cessation devices

Which smoking cessation device should you use, to help you stop smoking? Should you use nicotine gum or nicotine patches? Should you try to quit with the help of electronic cigarettes?

You should not use any, period.

When people use nicotine gum to help them stop smoking, all they do is change a nicotine delivery method. We are dealing with an addiction here. Our brains do not care which device you use, as long as they get their "dope". You are not addicted to the cigarette or smoking per se, you are addicted to the nicotine. You have to break the addiction, not support it with some other method of nicotine delivery. I always advise quitting cold turkey! Now that you understand the nature of addiction, it should not be a problem, so stay away from any devices, you do not need them and it will only slow you down!

Electronic cigarettes are gaining popularity, but they are far from being safe! Governments around the world are only now starting to regulate them. Electronic cigarettes are banned from usage in public places in many countries. They are relatively new and there is not enough evidence to label them safe. Studies show that vapor from electronic cigarettes contains cancer-causing agents. They are far from harmless devices some people think, or would like you to believe they are. Not so long ago, we though cigarettes are safe too.

You already have the best anti-smoking device and carry it around all the time. It is your brains! It is true; you are addicted to nicotine because of them, but the moment you "see the light", your brains will become your best friend, helping you beat the addiction. All it takes is a change of perspective.

Smoke the last cigarette IN YOUR LIFE!

You have to prepare mentally. Nicotine addiction is strong and it is not easy to quit smoking if you are not prepared. Most smokers can go without a cigarette for a few days, even weeks. Then the biggest mistake happens - they smoke a cigarette. Boom! They are addicted again. Do not think that you can only smoke one. You cannot. As soon as you do, your addiction is back.

After you quit smoking you can never, and that means NEVER smoke another cigarette in your life. Not even a single drag from your friend. Prepare yourself for that. Smoke another cigarette now, if you have to. Finish the open pack if you do not want to throw it away. But keep in mind that once you decide to quit smoking, it has to be final and you cannot smoke a single cigarette ever again.

Like an ex-alcoholic is always just one glass of alcohol away from returning to addiction, you will always be one cigarette away from becoming smoker and nicotine addict again. It might sound terrible right now, but you have my promise, the hard part will only last for a few weeks. After that, staying non-smoker will not require much effort from your side until finally, after a few months; it will not require ANY effort!

Manage cravings

Are you afraid to quit smoking, because you know that there will be times when you will experience cravings? You fear that there will be times, when you will not be able to resist the temptation. I had those fears, and I have yet to meet a smoker that doesn't.

There will be cravings after you stop smoking. It would be a blatant lie if I told you that you will experience none. The important thing to remember is, that you will experience only a few of them each day. You will not crave smoking 24/7. There will be more cravings in the first few days and then less with each passing day. The duration of cravings also changes with time. After a few days, each craving will last less than three minutes. The "only" thing you have to do is to resist smoking for a few minutes a day. It is not easy, but not that hard either. Just focus your thoughts on something else and they will pass.

You can experience cravings for a few months, but later on, they are very mild and irregular. After a few months, cravings last only a couple of seconds and are very ease to manage. You pass some place where you used to smoke and it brings up memories and induce a short craving. But at that time you will already know exactly how to reach. You will not panic. To tell you the truth, the only cravings that are somehow hard to manage are those in early weeks. They are more intense and last longer.

It is crucial, not to project early withdrawal symptoms into the future, believing you will always feel like you feel for the first few days or weeks.

That is the number one reason people fail to quit smoking - they give up to early.

They experience a few intense cravings for a few days and think it will always be like that. It happened to me too. I thought is just not worth it to go through all this nervousness and irritability. I was so nervous I did not know where to put my hands. My previous quitting attempts helped me through those early days. I already knew that the hardest part would be over soon. Still, minutes felt like hours and hours felt like days! Please, do not get scared. It will be over eventually and millions of people did it before you. Think of that. If they managed it, so will you. It will be tough for a few days, but at the end, it is all worth it thousand times over.

I feel sad, when I hear stories of individuals that made it to week three, and smoked a cigarette. They have been through the toughest part already and blew it. I wish I could show you how easy it will be to stay non-smoker after a months later. No more cravings, not even one.

Find support

Find someone that will help you through the process of becoming a non-smoker. This is a very important step. At times, it can make all the difference between you smoking and not smoking.

For my girlfriend and me, it was relatively easy. We both stopped at the same time so we supported each other. When I became weak, she reminded me of the reasons I decided to quit smoking. She supported me when I needed help. It does not take much. She didn't need to fight me, not to smoke. A gentle reminder here or there was enough. When she was in trouble, I gave her support. After a few months, she told me there were times when she almost slipped. It was enough to distract her for a few moments to avoid the "disaster".

The process of becoming a non-smoker is fairly long. That means that you will encounter various stressful situations during that time. When such time comes, you will think irrationally. Our brains are masters of deception so you will quickly find a reason to smoke a cigarette. You will suddenly feel it is just not worth suffering so much. It only takes one cigarette to for you to become addicted again. This is the main reason you need someone who can think clearly and will support you at this time of weakness.

It does not matter who that person is. It could be your best friend, a family member, a co-worker. It can be all of them. The more, the better. You can try to persuade one of your family members or one of your friends to quit smoking with you. That will significantly increase the chance of success for both.

Tell people around you that you are going to quit smoking and that you will need their support. Tell them that you will possibly think of smoking a cigarette and ask them to remind you of the reasons you decided to quit smoking. This should be enough for the craving to pass.

Change your habits

One of the most difficult things of quitting smoking are your habits and rituals. There are things and places that remind you of smoking and those places alone will induce a craving. Stay strong, this too shall pass!

For me, the hardest part were vacations. A bottle of beer in one hand, the cigarette in the other. I was terrified before I went on vacations for the first time after quitting smoking. But you know what, it was not that bad, not at all. I had a few cravings, but that was all. The next thing on my list was coffee. For a few weeks, every time I saw a cup of coffee, I had a minor craving. Again, first few cravings were more intense, then less and less so. Nothing to terrible and certainly manageable.

My girlfriend had her own little rituals connected to smoking. One of those rituals was when she was cleaning the apartment. After finishing half the apartment, she would take a break, smoked a cigarette and then continued with cleaning. When she saw vacuum cleaner, her brains saw cigarettes and that in turn, induces craving. This is a habit and we humans are creatures of habit. To make it easier, she replaced a habit of smoking with a habit of drinking coffee. Now when she is done with cleaning the apartment, she sits down and enjoys a cup of coffee.

You have your own places and rituals where you are used to smoking. After you quit smoking, you have to go through each of those rituals and not smoke. The first time it will be hard, the next time it will be a lot easier. Break or replace your habits. This has nothing to do with the physical addiction. We are used to doing various things and smoking at the same time, so we develop a habit. It is therefore normal that our brains expect us to smoke when we do those same things. Nevertheless, your brains will also get used to doing those same things without smoking. Get rid of unhealthy habits first, and then develop healthy ones.

How not to gain weight

People fear that they will gain weight after quitting smoking. It depends on how you do it and how you prepare for it. I did not gain a single pound after quitting and neither did my girlfriend. To tell you the truth, we both lost some weight. That has probably more to do with us becoming more active than smoking itself. Anyway, there is no direct relationship between quitting smoking and gaining weight. So if you want the scale to stay where it is, take one advice:

Stay away from unhealthy food!

Some people gain weight after quitting smoking because they are nervous and seek comfort in food. Do not do that! Food will not give you the comfort you seek, when you miss smoking! Nothing but nicotine, can replace nicotine! It does not matter if you eat sweets or hamburgers instead of smoking. You will still experience cravings; you will still experience withdrawal symptoms. You will still be irritable and nervous for a few days. If you have to chew on something to calm down, get some carrots or some other healthy snacks.

You should not gain any weight, but prepare up-front. Throw away all the chocolates, chips and candies. Stash your cabinet with fruits, almonds, cashews and pistachios. Better yet - prepare your sneakers. That is sneakers, not Snickers!

Which gets us to the next topic.

Start exercising

Move! Get out of the house! Go for a walk! No matter which activity you choose, it will help you greatly.

My girlfriend and I started with long walks. We spent half of that time talking about cigarettes, walking for miles without even realizing how far we went. We discussed all kinds of things related to smoking, how many cravings each of us had, how we manage them. You do not need to ignore cravings and it is perfectly fine if you talk about them with whomever is present at the time. Cravings are a part of breaking the addiction.

Back to exercising. Why is it so important for you? For starters, scientist proved that exercising releases endorphins — "hormones" that make you feel happy. It is the same hormone that is released when you have sex or when you eat chocolate.

You like both, don't you? After you quit smoking, you need to "entertain" your brains. You have to deliver them something that feels good, and endorphins are exactly what they need at that time - lots of them!

Exercise is healthy, takes your time and mind of smoking and it makes you happy! It also improves your mood and raises your energy level. What more do you wish for. There are many other benefits besides those listed. The important thing for you is to incorporate regular exercise in your daily or weekly schedule, no matter which activity you choose.

Start slowly at the beginning. Your lungs and heart needs time to improve. If you are not in a good shape, I suggest you start with walks. Then, as you get better, increase the speed of walking and later, do it uphill. You can also start jogging. This is all it takes to keep yourself in a good shape. There is no need to run marathons, although nothing wrong with that too.

When it comes to exercising, it is important to set goals and then work towards them. Keep a log or a diary. That way you can track your improvements. You can do it the old style, with a piece of paper and a pen, or create a computer. Track how many minutes you spent exercising daily and weekly, the distance you covered. After reaching your goal, set another one and repeat.

Be careful! You can become addicted to exercising, whether it be running, cycling or working out. You do not want your next book to be: How to get rid of exercising addiction... Just kidding of course, do it as much as you like!

Chapter 14: How Your Smoking Affects Others

It is well-known that smoking is extremely bad for your health and is not advised. It has always been well-publicized that breathing in the smoke of others can also be hazardous to one's health.

What exactly is secondhand smoke?

There are two different kinds of secondhand smoke, both of which come from the smoke exhaled by smokers. First, there is the mainstream smoke, which is the obvious smoke that a smoker actually exhales, and the other is sidestream smoke, which is the smoke that comes from the end of the actual cigarette.

Although secondhand may seem harmless, that could not be further from the truth. It contains thousands of chemicals including a number of deadly elements such as ammonia, arsenic, hydrogen cyanide, and so on. Many of these elements are proven to be toxic, dangerous, and known to cause cancer.

The risks of secondhand smoke

There are a multitude of risks that people are susceptible to when they are in the vicinity of those that smoke, including:

-Breathing problems

-Chest infections

-Coughing

-Heart disease

-Sore throats

- Cancer

- Asthma-triggering an attack for asthmatics and also the risk of others developing asthma

This proves that second-hand smoke cannot just make an impact on a person's future but it is also capable of causing problems for that person immediately. Of particular note is the fact that second-hand smoke can affect someone's sports ability or performance with regards to how physically active they can be.

How to avoid secondhand smoke

You more than likely know someone that smokes, whether this is a family member, a person that you socialize with or a work colleague. Regardless of whether or not you smoke, or you just hang out with someone that does for a prolonged period of time, the fact remains that it is not healthy to breathe in any kind of tobacco smoke. Occasional exposure, even short-term, will at some point takes a toll on your body and could lead to a severe illness.

If you are the smoker, then you must try to give this up. Although giving up is not easy because of smoking being such a highly addictive activity, one thing is for sure and this is that you can do it. Not only are you worth it, but also those around you are worth it too.

There are so many benefits that you can obtain from giving up smoking: not only will you look and feel better than ever before, but also you will be far wealthier and have money which you can then use to treat yourself. It is possible that you may never have realized the devastating effects your smoke is having on you and your loved ones. Maybe realizing that by quitting, you are protecting those loved ones that are dear to you, could be just the thing you need to reinforce your determination and willpower and quit smoking for good.

If you are not a smoker but do know smokers then ask them politely to observe the following habits:

1. Only ever smoke outside away from other people particularly children and expectant mothers. As smoke lingers in the air hours after the cigarette is put out, someone that smokes indoors is subjecting others to breathe and inhale their smoke too.

2. The smoker should make a habit of not smoking when they have other people in their vehicle or if they are a passenger. Exhaling the smoke through an open window does little if anything to reduce the exposure to other individuals.

There has been a lot of research and studies carried out particularly recently on the subject of second-hand smoke and its dangers and this is why it's so important for those who do smoke to be sensible and respect the wishes of others.

Smokers choose to light their next cigarette, and non-smokers should have a choice too.

The new laws and reforms that have come into place over the past years regarding smoking have made it far easier for non-smokers, and gives them protection to ensure they are not subjected to second-hand smoke.

If you are a non-smoker, stand up for your rights and reinforce your rights regarding second-hand smoke. In the same breath if you are a smoker understand the effects that this habit of yours is having on those around you, and just be considerate. There is absolutely no doubt that by eliminating second-hand smoke from your life, you will keep your body much healthier. This could be just the thing to help someone you love think about kicking the habit for good.

Chapter 15: Why People Continue To Smoke Even When There Are Aware Of The Dangers Associated With It?

In the last issue we talked about what happens after you finally quit smoking. In this issue we are going to talk about why people continue to smoke even when there are aware of the dangers associated with it.

Most people are well aware of the dangers and disadvantages that are caused by smoking, still they continue to smoke and there are many that are never able to completely give up the habit.

There are many chain smokers who smoke 30 cigarettes a day not because of their body has a real craving for nicotine, but because they have become habitual. They need it to satisfy their habit.

An interesting reality is that when we continue smoking the effect of drug lessens but arouses a psychological need for more doses to increase effects. This is how; we become mere puppets of our own body. It is not an easy habit to kick.

That leads us to believe that smoking is a problem of mind and not of body!

Have you ever wondered how we can make our body understand that we can't smoke for several hours at a time while at work or on a long ride or airplane flight? If we can make it for those long periods of time then why can't we just quit?

The answer is habit has an environmental trigger. It switches on when we pick up the phone, sit in a chair, after meals, with a drink etc.

Smokers truly believe that smoking gives them pleasure. This is because of daily habit and quitting a bad habit is much more difficult than becoming free from nicotine addiction.

Some studies show that quitting is a fairly easy task if you can get your mind to cooperate. Hypnotherapy has been found an effective means by which some people can remove environmental triggers from their thought process and quit smoking more easily.

Chapter 16: Beating Addiction

In this section I describe the method that I used to tackle my addiction. It started with asking myself, that given all that we have described so far, what on earth was I doing still smoking.

I determined that the logical sane part of me must be being over powered by something. That something was the addiction and I hated the feeling that I was an addict with all the negative connotations that implies.

I decided to personify that addiction as a monster / demon / beast that had infiltrated my body in order to slowly destroy me.

Personifying the monster meant that I had somebody/something to battle against. It wasn't me, it was an intruder (akin to a virus in a computer) and it was smart. It was going to use every trick in its armoury to stay firmly in control and lodged within my body.

I know that this might seem a little odd but I want you to accept that this is what has happened to you. Now, I want you to visualise and name this intruder. If you name it, you accept that it exists. If you give it a name you can, if this works for you, opt to give it one that starts to denigrate its status. Alternatively you can give it a strong name in recognition of its force over you.

Name it and, if it helps you, sketch it.

This beast inside you is tough, very tough and it is extremely cunning. It will lie to you and deceive you. It will let you think you are winning and then come back at you when you least expect it. So what we need to do is use the full strength of our logical side to overcome it.

One final thought on this. You will need to make and keep your desire to defeat the beast stronger than the perceived pleasure you get from smoking. At some stage in the quit plan the beast will tell you that you like smoking ('I enjoy a cigarette, it calms me, I actually like smoking') and you may be persuaded that those thoughts actually outweigh all the negatives that we've already outlined. They don't by the way.

So to win this battle (and it is a battle) make your desire to out-smart, purge, slay the beast your primary goal for the next few weeks.

The Commitment

So you've decided you are going to beat this addiction monster. You are going to be a wealthier, healthier, cooler smoker who doesn't smoke.

I now want you to think about this scenario. Who in the world would you least like to tell that you failed to give up smoking? The one person (or group if you prefer) that it would make you cringe to have to admit that you were not able to give up the habit.

Before you start the quit programme, I am going to ask you to tell them in the most emphatic way possible that you are giving up smoking and that you are deadly serious this time.

Don't hedge your bets here and choose a soft option. If you hedge now you will greatly reduce your chances of success. You need to choose the most powerful ally. I use the word ally deliberately because when you think of giving up the fight you need to play out how you are going to feel about telling this person you've failed.

Chapter 17: You've Quit!

My last diary entry was 289. This is how many days I had been cigarette free and I was certain at that point that the technique had worked. I no longer felt the need to reward myself with a daily achievement number and my life as a nonsmoker was established. I was at this point able to go to parties and get drunk, if I chose to, without the spectre of slipping back into smoking. No longer did I feel as though I had to avoid other smokers or those situations where smoking had previously accompanied the occasion. The sheer euphoric pleasure of knowing I was no longer a slave to nicotine cannot be over emphasised. Remember this is the story of how I quit. It worked for me, a weak willed person who absolutely loved smoking for many years. There are many other self-help guides out there who promise quick results and secret techniques to get you to quit and while these may be completely valid my method is based on actual experience, and it works. I have met several people over the years, and I am sure you have too, who have simply quit! I applaud and admire them but I think they are few and far between, the rest of us mortals need a bit of help, I certainly did, and I hope that by sharing my success story I have been able to help you too.

My smoking related morning cough and rasping laugh had disappeared and my sense of smell had returned. Intrinsically linked with smell is the ability to taste food again. Combined with the removal of nicotine's apatite suppressing properties and I found I had started to put on a few pounds. As mentioned earlier, this was not an aspect of quitting that I feel is worth concentrating on whilst going through the quitting process.

You will probably discover, as I did, a new zest for life and an increase in energy levels. For me I waited until the nicotine addiction had been overcome before concentrating on the side effects. You can after all deal with these far more easily than you can deal with the potentially lethal effects of smoking.

In my case I chose to take up my childhood hobby of cycling. I bought myself a second hand cycle and over the subsequent months managed to improve from an asthmatic half mile slog to enjoyable brisk twenty mile country rides. I am still very slow but I enjoy the energy and weight control it has brought into my life. I feel my lungs with clean air and feel the blood coursing through my veins. I have also completed four marathon length walks for charity, something that I could not ever have contemplated as a smoker.

These again are my outlets, and I am not saying you too should rush out and buy a set of Lycra or hiking shoes, but do something. Part of your epiphany will be to add a new dimension to your life. If it helps control your weight, if that is becoming an issue, then great, but it just needs to be something you can be proud of, something you enjoy that challenges you and is perhaps something you could not have done as a smoker. Learn to ride a horse, go swimming, join a rambling club, learn to sail, dance, take up yoga the possibilities are endless, just do something new, you will be so glad that you did.

I sincerely hope that you enjoyed this little story of how I quit smoking and that it will inspire you to do the same. Remember to be kind to yourself and involve your friends and family in your journey. You really are much stronger and more capable than you think. I did it, so can you.

I am so pleased that you have made it to this point, you are amazing, well done. If you need or a reminder of the key points of how I and hopefully you quit I thought it would be useful to give a brief checklist for you, remember 'fail to prepare; prepare to fail':-

Visualise cigarettes as a friend or relative you loved but who has passed away and they are not coming back into your life.

Choose the day you quit, Day Zero, very carefully.

Let everyone know you are quitting, the day and that it will be for life. Ask them to support you.

Actively and consciously reduce the number of cigarettes you smoke over the month prior to Day Zero.

Purchase a physical paper diary.

Make a list in your diary of every reason you want to quit - put HEALTH at the top of the list.

Purchase Nicotine Replacement Therapy but not a Vape or E-Cigarette - in my case micro-tabs, also stock up on a 'comforter' - strong mints (Fishermen's Friends were mine) etc.

Remove all smoking paraphernalia from everywhere. Lighters, ashtrays, matches etc.

Clean everywhere just prior to quitting. Your home, car and of course yourself!

The night before Day Zero enjoy and say farewell to your last ever cigarette. Say goodbye to you as a smoker.

Early cravings will come thick and fast as nicotine loses its grip, when they do use your NRT liberally whenever required. Combine it with your comforter to give a continuous distraction.

Note each successful day in your diary, this will build into an achievement record that you just won't want to restart.

Reward yourself frequently for your achievements.

Avoid trigger situations, change your routine and habits.

Do not worry about food cravings during the early stages, you can deal with these after you have broken the addiction.

Actively seek the support of friends and family throughout your journey.

Do not drink alone, your guard will be down and nicotine is a very manipulative and powerful drug.

Remember you will still be vulnerable for a long time after Day Zero. Do not ever be tempted to think you can dip in and out of smoking, you are now a nonsmoker and cigarettes are dead to you.

Take up a new activity or hobby when you feel mentally and physically able to.

Stick to this schedule, as I did, and I can assure you that you can do it. Most importantly is that you do not waiver no matter what. Quitting is partly beating the chemical addiction and this is the biggest hurdle to overcome but the longer and perhaps trickier challenge is ridding yourself of the psychological addiction.

By preparing correctly and anticipating what is to come you can beat both of the chains that tie you to this ridiculous and lethal habit.

Chapter 18: Instructions To Follow To Avoid Those Thing That Make You Want To Smoke

1. Alcoholic Drink:

Almost all the smokers engage in the habit of smoking when they are taking alcoholic drink. If you're such a person, you may opt for drink that does not contain alcholic content or better still find a place where smoking is not allowed and have your drink. You can chew cocktail or you can suck on a straw and try snacks as alternatives.

2. Surrounded by other people who are also smokers:

If your family member, friends and the people you work with in the office all smoke around you, it will be so hard to quit the habit or avoid going back when you've quitted. Tell them you seriously want to quit and they will not smoke when you're inside a car with them or when you're taking coffee with them during break at work. In the place you work look for a person who does not smoke and have your break with such person or you can decide to do other things like taking a brief walk, reading a book, drawing etc.

3. Whenever smokers are approaching the end of their meal:

Several people who smokes indulge in the act whenever they are wrapping up their food and the hope of giving up this habit will be very slim. But, what you can do to stop this, is replacing that moment after you've eating with another thing like taking a small quantity of fruit, desert that are good, chewing gum or taking a chocolate and biscuit. When you do this daily you'll forget to light that cigarette after meal with time.

Managing symptoms that comes with nicotine withdrawal

The moment you no longer smoke, they are various physical symptoms your body will experience when your body withdraws from nicotine. When your body is withdrawing from nicotine it happens quickly, this normally start within 60 minutes after the last cigarette and going up from there two to three days later. These withdrawal symptoms may last for some days to several weeks, but the way it happens to one person is different from the way it happens to another person.

Some known nicotine withdrawal symptoms are:

Cravings to smoke cigarette

They will be irritation, the person will be frustrated and angry

The person will be Anxious and nervous

The person will find it hard to concentrate

The person will be restless

The person will always feel hungry to eat food

The person will experience headaches

Insomnia

Tremors

The person will be coughing uncontrollably

Fatigue

He will have stomach upset and constipation

The person will be depressed

Heart rate will be immensely reduced

Even though all the above symptoms that occur when withdrawing from nicotine are not pleasant, but it is worthy to know that all the above symptoms are not permanent but temporal. As the toxins are being removed from their body, they will feel better and strong in some weeks. For now tell your family and friend that you're not your usual self again and ask them to understand your point of view.

Chapter 19: Nutrition And Quitting Smoking-Managing Weight Gain After Quitting And The Essential Quitters Diet

One of the most ignored aspects of quitting smoking is nutrition. Most smokers who are on the path of quitting may find that their nutrition is inhibitive or counterproductive to quitting. Let us get a bit real. When you quit smoking or a few weeks into your quitting plan, the urge for nicotine is bound to be at an all time high at one point or the other. Drinking a dozen pots of coffee is a very common occurrence in quitters. One of the most important things that you can do to help in your quitting endeavor is to avoid coffee or caffeinated drinks. Coffee multiplies the cravings and makes it extremely hard for you to say no to a cigarette. If you always have a cup of coffee in the morning, I suggest you change this to green tea or a fruit smoothie. A study conducted by Duke University indicated that fruits, vegetables and dairy products make cigarette smoke taste terrible, while red meat, alcohol and coffee make the smoke much tastier. A few weeks before you start your journey to stop smoking, drink many non-caffeinated drinks such as water and eat lots of fruits and vegetables. Continue this even after you have quit, and your cravings for cigarettes and nicotine will subside greatly.

Foods rich in vitamin C are also ideal for a person who is quitting smoking. Vitamin C can be found in fruits such as oranges, lime, lemons and guavas. Vitamin C diminishes the urge to smoke and makes it easier for you to cope with withdrawal symptoms like nicotine cravings. An effective way of using vitamin C to help you fight the craving is by eating slices of orange whenever you feel the cigarette cravings building up. To get rid of the urge to smoke, you can put a pinch of salt on the tip of your tongue to help satiate the urge. Alternatively, you can opt to eat salty snacks such as salted pickles.

Some of the reasons why most people are bound to gain weight after quitting are because cigarette smoking is an appetite suppressant. Thus, once you quit, your appetite will go back to normal, which means that you might start eating more food than you normally would when smoking. This is good since good appetite is an indication that the body is actively working to reverse the damages that smoking had inflicted on your body. In other instances, eating snacks is advised whenever the urge to smoke builds up. These two factors might cause a weight increase. However, do not give up since with a regular workout schedule, you do not need to worry about this. The best exercise for before and after quitting are all exercises that are geared towards increasing respiration and blood circulation in the body such as jogging and brisk walking.

The trick to keeping your weight in check after you have quit smoking is not to indulge in binge eating, as you will be tempted. If you were used to smoking in the morning and have now stopped, you will be tempted to eat to fill up the time that you would have otherwise used to smoke. If you feel that you must eat, eat only healthy foods such as nuts and fruits; carrots are also a very good alternative. After you quit smoking, you might experience some low blood sugar. It is advisable to consume foods that will gradually release sugar into your blood stream. Foods such as apricots and natural yoghurt are ideal.

Serotonin in your body helps deal with depression and foods that are high in serotonin will help you deal with some of the depression that might accompany your quitting plan. Foods that are essential for serotonin release into your body are turkey, fish and chicken. Another effect of quitting smoking is a decrease in concentration span. This is usually since nicotine has been shown to increase the concentration span of a user. To deal with this, you should consume proteins that have been found to be effective in helping you stay alert. These include egg whites, fish and beans.

In order to flush your body of the smoke toxins, you should drink more healthy fluids during quitting period and even after. Avoid alcohol and caffeine and instead opt for healthier drinks such as water, green tea and fresh fruit juice. A glass of warm milk before bed will help you feel relaxed and make you sleep better.

Another tip that I think is important when examining your diet is to listen to your body. Eat only when you are hungry and stop eating the moment you feel satisfied. This will make sure that you do not overeat and thus do not gain extra pounds. An effective trick to accomplish this is to divide your plate into three portions. The biggest portion, which should be half of your plate should be filled with vegetables, and a quarter of the rest of the plate should be filled with grains such as rice, while the remaining quarter should be filled with proteins. This method of diet control is called the plate method and it works like a charm. It ensures that your dietary intakes are balanced well and also ensures that you consume more vegetables.

Chapter 20: Focus On The Benefits Of Smoking (Hint: There Are No Benefits).

"The pessimist complains about the wind; the optimist expects it to change; the realist adjusts the sails." William Arthur Ward

People who try to quit often focus on the benefits of not smoking or the harms of smoking, which is a different side of the same coin. But that is not where the focus should be when you are trying to quit. The focus should be squarely on thinking about and understanding the **benefits of smoking**, or the lack thereof. Give yourself a few moments or a day to think about what you believe are the benefits of smoking—I mean really think about it.

There are many things that a smoker could come up with as the purported "benefits" that he or she gets in smoking. One of the most common things smokers say when asked why they smoke is "smoking relaxes me" or "smoking relieves my stress." But, as you know, nicotine is a stimulant. Smoking raises your heart rate and blood pressure. It makes you "wired," albeit in mild and ineffective manner.

A smoker may still insist that smoking provides "relaxation" or "relief" from stress, but the smoker may be misattributing the effects of the cigarette smoke with his or her smoking routine. For example, the routine of going on a "smoke break" may actually provide relaxation or stress relief, but that's not from the nicotine stick. Rather, the relaxation comes from the fact that the smoker is on a break. Next time you want to take a "smoke break," by all means, go for a break, but without smoking. Instead, go outside and take a deep breath. Even in the most polluted of cities, a deep breath of air outside will be more refreshing and relaxing than taking a puff of the toxic, carcinogenic cigarette smoke.

Like in a "smoke break," a form of relaxation may come from situations in which smokers find themselves when they are smoking, but they are giving the undeserved credit to the cigarette smoke. This applies to virtually every "trigger" situations. If one of your trigger situation is going #2 in the bathroom, that situation relieves stress certainly—but the relief is coming by way of (or into) the toilet, not by way of cigarette smoke going into your mouth, throat, and lungs.

Also remember that the supposed "stress" to be relieved is created by smoking cigarettes. Smokers are stressed when they want to smoke but cannot, for one reason or another. The time for the meeting to end, or the "smoke break" to come, or the class to finish, or the flight to land, or numerous other non-smoking situation to end cannot come soon enough for devoted smokers, so that they can go outside, take out their cancer sticks, and take a puff to feed the nicotine beggar inside them. Such situations create tremendous stress in smokers—stress that nonsmokers never have to face. Nonsmokers are not antsy to go outside in freezing or raining weather to take a puff of toxic smoke.

Smoking provides neither relaxation nor relief from stress. If you believe there are any benefits to smoking, give it some thought and think about the reasons. You will soon come to an understanding that you smoke because you are addicted to the nicotine smoke, and not because there are any benefits to smoking. It is very important that you come to this understanding—that you truly know in your heart and mind that there are no benefits to smoking. A cigarette is not your stress reliever, a relaxation aid, or your "friend." A cigarette is simply a cancer stick that you have been duped into taking day-in-and-day-out because you have been conditioned to do so over time, and re-enforced to do so through the nicotine chemical in the cigarette. The act of smoking is a disease, disease of the mind. Accept this fact. Once you accept this truth, stopping smoking is easy.

Chapter 21: A New Kind Of Cleaning

When I was trying to quit, I found out that if I went swimming or went to the beach the urge reduced drastically but few minutes in my clothes or in my room and boom it was back with full force.

I actually thought I was going crazy until I asked my therapist and she thankfully solved the puzzle and gave a solution that helped me so much.

If you are an avid smoker then there is a chance that the cigarette smell is embedded in every piece of clothing you own, that also includes your furniture and upholstery in your car.

Sadly some detergents don't fully mask the smell and in fact like I learnt perfumes won't fully mask it so here is where the really experienced dry cleaners come in, I must tell you that this might cost you some money but the reward will really outstrip the money spent and ensure you don't keep spend money on cigarettes.

I remember leaving my house to stay with my mum so every single place can be cleaned and when I came back my house became my fortress of strength and it smelled fresh and the urge to smoke went down drastically because of this single action.

I recommend it to anyone that is serious about quitting but there is one thing though, even though we cleaned the house we left one remnant of dirt that is really important.

THE IMPORTANT REMNANT

When you are packing for the cleaning I need you to pack every ashtray that hopefully has cigarette remnant and put them in an air tight bag and put water in it and keep it somewhere for few days.

Go get it the next time you feel like smoking and stick your nose in and sniff and I promise you might just throw up and that second is the moment you will start hating cigarettes and once you start hating it you are on your way to sweet freedom.

Chapter 22: How To Deal With Weight Gain And Other Side Effects

Of the many dreaded side effects of quitting smoking, weight gain is the one that almost every person is worried about. Gaining weight is a result of your body getting up on its feet and restoring their proper functions. As your sense of smell and taste perform better, you enjoy your food more and eating becomes more pleasurable. And since an essential part of cleansing your body is a lot of fluid, swelling and bloating is also unavoidable.

Most people are concerned about gaining weight due to quitting so they take the heroic act of quitting and at the same time watching their weight. But as you may already have known by now, quitting is already a very hard feat in itself. If you quit while watching your weight, it will only make things harder for you. But good news for you, it's just hard if you don't have a plan, and luckily, you already know how to make a quitting plan. Chapter 5 has already given you useful tips to help you avoid gain weight, and in this chapter you will know more.

1. Plan your meals

One of the most effective ways of watchingyour weight is by planning your meals. Include in your meals a balanced amount of healthy foods, like fruits and vegetable, whole wheat grains, and lightly seasoned protein. When your cravings kick in, don't nibble sweet biscuits or junk foods, and just stick to fruits and vegetables.

2. Keep moving

Set a time in your schedule for exercise. It can be a jog in the park every morning or a trip to the gym every week, or just a few crunches and sit-ups. Like in Chapter 6, you must keep yourself busy with physical activity. If you are not doing anything, move about the house or the offices to burn some calories while at the same time distracting yourself.

3. Avoid alcohol

Another thing to avoid if you don't want to gain weight is alcohol. Not only does alcohol lower your inhibition and make you susceptible to smoking again, some alcoholic drinks also contain a lot of calories. So, it's best to avoid drinking alcohol as much as possible.

4. Time your quit date perfectly

You also have to set your quitting date in a strategic and appropriate time. Avoid quitting on holidays since food is abundant during this time, especially when you are at final point in your quitting process. Remember that food becomes even delicious at this point in your recovery.

Other than the list of withdrawal symptoms listed in Chapter 5, quitting smoking has other side effects. Although they are not as intolerable and distressing, it's still important to know about them and learn how to deal with them.

Two of these other side effects include itchiness and skin blemishes. You can experience itchiness in the skin as a withdrawal symptom, as caused by the restoration of the circulation of blood to the skin, which can be easily addressed by balms and creams. In addition, as your body flushes out toxins, some of these get excreted through your skin, causing the appearance of acnes and skin blemishes. Nothing to worry though since these will disappear as soon as the body's system is cleansed.

The important thing to take note of is that these other side effects, including all the withdrawal symptoms, will just pass. Be glad instead as they are positive signs that the body is recovering and fighting back. Remember, success is more rewarding when you have suffered to get it, and though the ride may be hard, it will all be worth your while.

Chapter 23: Cigarette Smoking Cessation Drug

There are some medications as well as therapies that are offered either over-the-counter at your neighborhood drug store or that could be recommended by your medical professional that could aid you quit smoking cigarettes which could likewise assist with the desires as well as various other issues connected with cigarette smoking cessation.

It aids to taper down the prompts to smoke that many cigarette smokers have in the very early days and also weeks after giving up, instead of eliminate them absolutely. By tapering the prompts progressively, cigarette smokers are a lot better able to manage them, instead of really feeling an assault of yearnings as well as various other troubles right away.

Keep in mind that pure nicotine gum must not be eaten like normal gum. Pure nicotine spots and also various other items additionally should be utilized properly to be efficient.

These are helps that are created to slowly taper down the quantity of pure nicotine in your system to make sure that you could slowly eliminate your yearnings.

When taking any one of these drugs or utilizing these items, you have to take care to utilize the suggested dose and also adhere to all instructions precisely.

Why it functions.

The nasal spray supplies pure nicotine extremely swiftly, as well as could be made use of to eliminate extreme yearnings sometimes of the day when the cigarette smoker is useded to having a cigarette, while the spot provides a smaller sized dose of pure nicotine to the body at a steadier price.

Bear in mind preventative measures.

Integrating items.

As well as naturally, maintain these items far from kids and also family pets. Also a percentage of pure nicotine from any one of these could damage children particularly; do not wait to call emergency situation solutions or Poisonous substance Control instantly if you believe that your kid has actually consumed any one of these items.

One more sort of smoking cigarettes cessation medication, bupropion (Zyban), additionally decreases food craving as well as drawback signs and symptoms, although it is not a pure nicotine substitute item. Bupropion is an antidepressant drug that is believed to aid individuals quit smoking cigarettes by simulating several of the results of tobacco on mind cells. Bupropion could be made use of along with pure nicotine substitute items; a number of researches suggest that the mix aids even more cigarette smokers gave up compared to either technique on its own.

Transdermal pure nicotine spots, gum, lozenges, sprays, and also inhalers are all kinds of pure nicotine substitute treatments.

NRT does not have these ingredients, the tar, or any one of these various other contaminants, as a result a cigarette smoker is not just able to give up slowly yet is permitting these toxic substances to be eliminated from their body instantly, which likewise aids stem their yearnings.

Pure nicotine substitute treatments (NRT).

The nasal spray and also inhaler kind of NRT are just offered with a prescription, however spots are gum are normally offered nonprescription.

Some that have actually weighed cigarette smokers for an extended period of time could wish to review with their medical professionals a combo of NRT items, as an example, utilizing the spot and also the gum could assist greater than merely one alone.

There are obviously various other medicines and also antidepressants that your physician could recommend that could assist soothe your anxiousness and also anxiety that's related to cigarette smoking, which could assist with your specific yearnings or various other problems. It is essential that you as well as your medical professional collaborate to locate merely the best option for you and also your circumstance.

Furthermore, it's believed that one of the most unsafe element of cigarettes is not the pure nicotine itself, however the tar as well as various other contaminants that are contributed to cigarettes which are developed by the chain reaction of burning.

Buspirone (BuSpar) is a depressant that looks reliable in assisting cigarette smokers take care of sensations of anxiousness arising from tobacco drawback.

NRT provides pure nicotine to the cigarette smoker's human brain in a much slower means compared to cigarettes do. When an individual breathes in a cigarette, pure nicotine gets in the lungs and after that takes a trip to the mind within secs, providing the "rush" that cigarette smokers pertain to yearn for.

When making use of NRT items, also those that are over the counter, you must be in touch with your doctor consistently. They will certainly inspect making certain the medication is functioning as it ought to and also will certainly look for undesirable adverse effects.

Adverse effects of these medicines could consist of:

Believe seriously regarding your family and friends as well as exactly what they could do to urge you to avoid brightening once more.

Some side results might be moderate, your medical professional might desire to suggest various other medicines to aid ease some of these signs and symptoms if they are serious. Once again, consistently be in touch with your physician on a regular basis as well as be straightforward concerning any type of negative effects or various other problems you are having.

An unique note for mamas.

Pure nicotine enters bust milk as well as might create troubles for nursing infants. Ladies that are nursing as well as intend to utilize cigarette smoking cessation medications could should quit nursing throughout therapy.

As consistently, remain in continuous call with your obstetrician or various other medical professional while breastfeeding as well as ensure you are following his/her referrals entirely.

queasiness.

throwing up.

serious discomfort in the tummy or abdominal area.

serious looseness of the bowels.

extreme lightheadedness.

fainting.

convulsions (seizures).

reduced high blood pressure.

quick, weak, or uneven heart beat.

hearing or vision troubles.

serious breathing issues.

serious watering of the mouth or salivating.

anxiety.

extreme frustration.

complication.

serious weak point.

Pure nicotine in any sort of kind must not be utilized while pregnant, as it might hurt the unborn child or trigger miscarriage. Ladies that could conceive must utilize reliable contraception while taking cigarette smoking cessation medications. Ladies that conceive while taking this medication must quit taking it promptly and also contact their doctors.

Conclusion

Thank you again for downloading this book!

I hope this book was able to help you to get your facts straight about what Smoking Addiction is and how to cure it.

The next step is to use the tips and strategies we've listed down all throughout this book and find a method that works for you. There can only be good things that come for those who quit smoking!

Thank you and good luck!

www.ingramcontent.com/pod-product-compliance
Lightning Source LLC
Chambersburg PA
CBHW071828080526
44589CB00012B/951